INTERMITTENT FASTING:
TRANSFORM YOUR BODY AND MIND

Lose weight, look younger, regulate your hormones, rejuvenate your cells, and boost your energy.

Discover the revolution that is transforming middle-aged people into the best version of themselves.

Ry Shimanski

Intermittent Fasting: Transform Your Body and Mind

Copyright © 2024 by Ry Shimanski

ISBN

Digital xxxxxxxxxxxxxxxxxxx

Print xxxxxxxxxxxxxxxxxxxxxxxxxxxx

All rights reserved.

This book is meant for educational, informational, and demonstration purposes only and is not offering medical advice or medical treatment. The information it contains is not intended to be used for self-diagnosis or to replace medical care. Always consult qualified healthcare providers for advice on medical issues. The information found within does not create a therapeutic relationship or guarantee better mental health or physical movement. Neither the author nor the publisher assumes any liability for any adverse consequences that may result from the information and material presented in this book.

No part of this book may be reproduced in any form or by any electronic or mechanical means, including information storage and retrieval systems, without written permission from the author, except for the use of brief quotations in a book review.

The digital version of this book requires a separate journal and art materials to make use of its experiential learning style.

TABLE OF CONTENTS

Introduction   **4**

Chapter 1   7

Chapter 2: Timing Over Tradition: The 16/8 Method Unpacked   14

Chapter 3: Setting the Stage for Success with Intermittent Fasting   30

Chapter 4: Night and Day: Syncing Fasting with Life's Rhythms   46

Chapter 5: Clarity and Vitality: Unveiling the Mind's Potential Through Fasting   63

Chapter 6: Adapt and Thrive: Intermittent Fasting Tailored for You   80

Chapter 7: Nourishing Your Fasting Lifestyle   95

Chapter 8: Smooth Sailing Through Fasting Challenges   112

Chapter 9: Mind Over Meal: Fostering a Positive Fasting Mindset   128

Conclusion   **146**

References   **148**

INTRODUCTION

For my wife and I, the journey to discovering intermittent fasting was, less a path we sought out and more a revelation that found us at our wits' end. After years of navigating the labyrinth of traditional diets, each promising the key to lasting health and vitality yet delivering nothing but fleeting results, we stumbled upon a concept so simple it felt almost revolutionary. This method is all about reconnecting with the code that is embedded within our ancient DNA. The modern systems of sustenance go against our natural design, put simply, human beings were not made to eat as much as we do. All over the planet, we are experiencing an awakening. People are becoming more in tune with their core vibration, and intermittent fasting is part of that momentum. When my wife and I first started intermittent fasting we noticed that we both felt like we were aligning with ourselves and everything around us, and that was in the first week. It's important to understand that your gut is connected to your health, your mental health and your overall wellbeing. Once you get your diet right then everything in your life will fall into place. Since doing this diet my wife and I have experienced profound shifts in our life. I remember looking at my wife thinking how beautiful she looked, she was beaming. Her skin and hair looked amazing, people commented that she had reversed the ageing process. Not only did she look good she felt good, her hormones balanced and she always seemed centred and happy, and the same went for me.

Introduction

Intermittent fasting, at its core, is an approach to eating that cycles between periods of fasting and eating. It's straightforward, adaptable, and, most importantly, rooted in the natural rhythms of our biology. Unlike the diet regimes that had failed us before, intermittent fasting didn't demand an overhaul of our diet but a recalibration of our eating schedule.

This book is born from a desire to share the transformative power of intermittent fasting, specifically tailored for the unique challenges and needs of middle-aged men and women. Our aim is not merely to alter dietary habits but to initiate a holistic transformation in how you approach health and well-being. We're here to provide a clear, manageable roadmap to integrating intermittent fasting into your life, complete with the science behind its benefits, practical advice for daily implementation, and strategies to navigate the bumps along the road.

Expect to find a blend of personal insights, scientific research, and actionable advice designed to guide you from the basics to more advanced facets of intermittent fasting. We've tailored this book to address the specific hurdles middle-aged individuals face, supported by real-life examples and evidence-based strategies.

It's common to encounter misconceptions about intermittent fasting, ranging from fears of muscle loss to dismissals of it as just another trend. We're here to dismantle these myths with facts, drawing on scientific studies and our journey. The benefits we've experienced—weight loss, enhanced focus, and a general uplift in health—are not just anecdotal but are supported by a growing body of research.

As you turn these pages, we invite you to keep an open mind. The beauty of intermittent fasting lies in its flexibility; it's not a one-size-fits-all solution but a framework that can be customised to fit your lifestyle, health goals, and personal preferences.

Consider this introduction an invitation to a journey of transformation. Whether you're new to intermittent fasting or looking to deepen your practice, this book is your companion to a healthier, more vibrant life.

Intermittent Fasting: Transform Your Body and Mind

Let's embark on this journey together, with the promise that by the final page, you'll be equipped to embrace intermittent fasting in a way that fits you best.

Welcome to a new chapter in your health and well-being and believe me this works! Let's begin.

Chapter 1

Intermittent Fasting:
Transform Your
Body and Mind

Intermittent Fasting: Transform Your Body and Mind

In a world inundated with dietary advice and the next big health trends, the sheer volume of information can be overwhelming, especially for those of us navigating the subtle yet impactful shifts that come with age. Amidst this sea of guidance, intermittent fasting emerges not as a fleeting trend but as a lifestyle adjustment grounded in both history and science. Its appeal lies not in drastic dietary restrictions but in the timing of meals, aligning with our bodies' natural rhythms and offering a refreshing simplicity in our approach to health and wellness.

The Science Behind Fasting and Age-Related Metabolic Shifts

As we age, our bodies undergo a myriad of changes, often subtle and unnoticed until their cumulative effects become apparent. One such change is the gradual slowdown of our metabolism. This deceleration is not just a number on a scale; it reflects a deeper shift in how our bodies process energy, affecting everything from weight management to energy levels. The reasons behind this shift are multifaceted, involving changes in muscle mass, hormonal fluctuations, and alterations in cellular function.

Enter intermittent fasting, a practice that, rather than focusing on what to eat, reorients our attention to when we eat. This approach has shown promise in nudging our metabolism toward more youthful efficiency. By cycling between periods of eating and fasting, intermittent fasting does more than just limit calorie intake—it sparks a metabolic recalibration. During fasting periods, our bodies, in the absence of new energy sources from food, turn to stored fat for energy. This process not only aids in weight management but also kick-starts other metabolic improvements.

One notable benefit of intermittent fasting is its impact on insulin sensitivity. Insulin, a hormone produced by the pancreas, plays a critical role in regulating blood sugar levels. As insulin sensitivity improves, our cells become better able to respond to insulin, efficiently using glucose from our blood for energy. This enhancement can lead to reduced blood sugar levels, lowering the risk of type 2 diabetes—a condition that becomes increasingly common with age. The implications of improved insulin sensitivity extend beyond diabetes prevention, touching on overall metabolic health and vitality.

Moreover, intermittent fasting has been linked to the prevention of age-related diseases. Studies have shown that the practice can have protective effects against conditions like Alzheimer's disease and cardiovascular disease. For instance, the process of autophagy, a cellular "clean-up" mechanism activated during fasting, helps clear out damaged cells and regenerate newer, healthier ones, playing a role in preventing neurodegenerative diseases. Similarly, the positive effects of intermittent fasting on heart health, including improvements in blood pressure and cholesterol levels, contribute to a reduced risk of heart disease.

The intersection of intermittent fasting and age-related metabolic shifts presents a compelling case for considering this lifestyle adjustment. By aligning our eating patterns with our bodies' natural rhythms, we can support our metabolic health, enhance insulin sensitivity, and mitigate the risk of chronic diseases, laying the foundation for a healthier, more vibrant middle age and beyond.

1.3 Debunking Myths: What Intermittent Fasting Is and Isn't

In the landscape of health and wellness, intermittent fasting stands as a beacon of simplicity amidst a sea of complex diet regimens. However, its simplicity does not shield it from common misconceptions that can cloud its true nature and benefits. As we peel back the layers of myth surrounding intermittent fasting, we find a practice that is both adaptable and rooted in our biology, not a one-size-fits-all solution but a flexible framework designed to enhance our health and well-being.

Myth: Intermittent fasting is starvation

One of the most pervasive myths equates intermittent fasting with starvation, a misunderstanding that not only misrepresents the practice but also ignores its foundational principles. Starvation occurs in the absence of essential nutrients over extended periods, leading to detrimental health effects. Intermittent fasting, by contrast, is a structured approach to eating that alternates between periods of fasting and periods of eating. This pattern does not deprive the body of necessary nutrients but rather changes the timing of intake, allowing the body to enter periods of fasting that are natural and, importantly, manageable. When done correctly, intermittent fasting leads to a state where the body efficiently uses stored energy, far from the harmful effects associated with starvation.

Myth: Fasting leads to muscle loss

Another concern often voiced is the fear that intermittent fasting will lead to muscle loss, an understandable apprehension for anyone looking to maintain or improve their physical fitness. However, evidence suggests that when intermittent fasting is paired with resistance training, muscle mass can be preserved and even increased. The key lies in the body's response to fasting; by altering energy sources, fasting prompts the body to burn fat for fuel. Moreover, fasting has been shown to increase levels of human growth hormone, which plays a vital role in muscle growth and maintenance. Adequate protein intake during eating periods and consistent resistance training are crucial components that help ensure muscle mass is not only preserved but enhanced.

Myth: Intermittent fasting works the same for everyone

The notion that intermittent fasting offers a universal solution is a myth that overlooks the rich tapestry of human diversity. Our bodies respond to fasting in varied ways, influenced by factors such as age, gender, health status, and lifestyle. For instance, someone with a highly active lifestyle may find a shorter fasting window more compatible with their energy demands, while others may thrive on longer fasts. Recognizing this diversity is crucial; it underscores the importance of customising the fasting plan to fit the individual's unique needs and goals. Tailoring the approach allows for a more enjoyable and sustainable practice, ensuring that intermittent fasting enhances rather than disrupts one's life.

Myth: Fasting is too difficult to maintain

At first glance, intermittent fasting might seem like a daunting lifestyle adjustment, particularly for those accustomed to regular meal patterns. However, its adaptability makes it a feasible and sustainable change for many. Transitioning to intermittent fasting doesn't necessitate an abrupt overhaul but can be approached gradually. Starting with a shorter fasting window and slowly extending its duration allows the body and mind to adapt without undue stress. Additionally, focusing on nutrient-dense foods during eating periods can help satiate hunger and provide sustained energy, making fasting periods more manageable. Flexibility in adjusting fasting windows to accommodate social events or changes in routine further enhances its sustainability, making intermittent fasting a viable long-term lifestyle adjustment rather than a transient dietary experiment.

As we navigate through the misconceptions surrounding intermittent fasting, it becomes clear that it's true essence lies not in rigid dietary restrictions but in a flexible, adaptable approach to eating that honours our body's natural rhythms. By debunking these myths, we shed light on the potential of intermittent fasting to enhance our health and well-being, offering a path that considers our individual needs and lifestyles.

1.6 Intermittent Fasting and Autophagy: Renewing Your Body

Autophagy, a term derived from the Greek words for "self" and "eating," is a biological process that plays a crucial role in maintaining our health at the cellular level. It's our body's way of cleaning the house - during autophagy, cells break down and remove damaged proteins and organelles, effectively clearing debris and recycling parts for new cell formation. This process is vital for cellular repair and regeneration, contributing to the body's ability to fight off diseases and age-related degeneration.

Intermittent fasting has a direct relationship with autophagy, acting as a switch that activates this cellular cleaning process. When we fast, the decrease in insulin levels and the increase in norepinephrine signal our cells to begin autophagy. Essentially, the fasting state puts our cells in a stress mode, prompting them to start cleaning and repairing to optimise efficiency. This is akin to what happens when we declutter our homes; by removing what's no longer useful, we make room for new, functional items. Similarly, autophagy removes cellular debris and makes way for new, healthy cells.

The benefits of autophagy extend far beyond simple cellular cleanup. Enhanced autophagy, triggered by intermittent fasting, has been linked to increased longevity and a reduction in the risk of many diseases. For example, by removing damaged cells that can lead to inflammation, autophagy plays a role in preventing inflammatory diseases and certain cancers. Moreover, the removal of faulty parts within cells can prevent neurodegenerative diseases such as Alzheimer's and Parkinson's, which are associated with the accumulation of protein aggregates. Autophagy also supports metabolic health by regulating insulin sensitivity, which is crucial for preventing diabetes and obesity.

To maximise the benefits of autophagy while adhering to an intermittent fasting regimen, it's essential to balance fasting with nutritional needs. This balance ensures that, while the body enters a state conducive to autophagy during fasting periods, it also receives the nutrients required for optimal health during eating windows. Here are some guidelines to achieve this balance:

- Prioritise nutrient-dense foods: When you do eat, focus on foods rich in vitamins, minerals, and antioxidants. These nutrients support cellular health and can enhance the benefits of autophagy. Think colourful fruits and vegetables, lean proteins, healthy fats, and whole grains.

- Stay hydrated: Proper hydration is essential for all bodily processes, including autophagy. Drinking plenty of water helps remove toxins from the body and supports cellular function.

- Consider the timing of your meals: Aligning your eating windows with your body's natural circadian rhythms can further enhance autophagy. Eating during daylight hours and fasting at night align with our body's natural inclinations for processing and resting, respectively.
- Incorporate physical activity: Exercise, much like fasting, can induce autophagy. Combining intermittent fasting with regular, moderate exercise can amplify the process of cellular renewal and repair.
- Listen to your body: Adjust your fasting schedule and dietary choices based on how you feel. If a particular pattern of intermittent fasting leaves you feeling depleted, consider adjusting the length of your fasting windows or the composition of your meals.

By understanding and leveraging the relationship between intermittent fasting and autophagy, we can tap into our body's innate ability to renew itself. This process of cellular decluttering and renewal is a powerful tool in our quest for longevity and disease prevention, offering a pathway to a healthier, more vibrant life. By balancing our fasting practices with mindful nutrition and lifestyle choices, we support our body's natural processes for maintaining optimal health at the cellular level.

Chapter 2: Timing Over Tradition: The 16/8 Method Unpacked

Chapter 2: Timing Over Tradition: The 16/8 Method Unpacked

Imagine your body as a high-performance vehicle. Just as premium fuel can optimise a car's efficiency, the timing of your fuel intake can do wonders for your body. Enter the 16/8 intermittent fasting method, a powerful yet straightforward tool that redefines not what you fuel your body with, but when. This approach has the potential to recalibrate your body's metabolic processes, akin to fine-tuning a car's engine for peak performance.

Overview of the 16/8 Method

The 16/8 method, often hailed as the gateway to intermittent fasting, divides the day into two segments: a 16-hour fasting window and an 8-hour eating window. Think of it as giving your body a daily "rest period" from digesting food, allowing it to focus on other essential maintenance tasks, like repairing cells and burning stored fat. It's the simplicity of this method that makes it so appealing. There's no need to count calories meticulously or follow a strict diet. Instead, you eat your daily meals within an 8-hour window that fits your lifestyle, then fast for 16 hours.

Benefits Specific to the 16/8 Method

- Weight Management: By reducing your eating window, you naturally limit your calorie intake without the need to obsess over every bite. This can lead to a gradual, sustainable weight loss.

- Improved Insulin Sensitivity: Fasting for 16 hours gives your body a break from producing insulin, which can help reduce your risk of type 2 diabetes.

- Enhanced Mental Clarity: Many, including my wife and I, report a boost in focus and cognitive function during the fasting state, potentially due to increased production of brain-derived neurotrophic factor (BDNF).

- Convenience: This method easily integrates into most lifestyles, making it a sustainable choice for long-term health benefits.

How to Start the 16/8 Method

Starting the 16/8 method can be as simple as skipping breakfast or moving dinner earlier. Here's a step-by-step guide to ease into it:

1. Choose Your Eating Window: Start by deciding on an 8-hour window that fits your daily routine. For many, this means eating between noon and 8 p.m.
2. Gradually Increase Fasting Time: If jumping straight into a 16-hour fast feels daunting, begin by fasting for 12 hours and gradually extend the fasting window by an hour every few days.
3. Stay Hydrated: Drink plenty of water during the fasting period to help suppress hunger and keep you hydrated.
4. Listen to Your Body: It's normal to feel hungrier than usual or a bit sluggish when you first start fasting. These feelings should subside as your body adjusts.

Tailoring the 16/8 Method to Your Life

The beauty of the 16/8 method lies in its flexibility. Here are some ways to adapt it to your needs:

- Adjust the Eating Window: If you're an early riser and prefer breakfast, shift your eating window to an earlier time, such as 7 a.m. to 3 p.m.
- Incorporate Nutrient-Dense Foods: During your eating window, focus on whole, nutrient-rich foods to maximise energy and satiety.
- Combine with Other Healthy Habits: Pair fasting with regular exercise and quality sleep to enhance its benefits.
- Social and Work Life: Plan social events and work commitments around your eating window when possible. If an event falls outside your window, consider shifting your eating window for that day.

Chapter 2: Timing Over Tradition: The 16/8 Method Unpacked

Visual Element: Interactive Quiz *Find Your Ideal 16/8 Fasting Window* This quiz helps you determine the best eating window based on your daily routine, sleep schedule, and social habits. By answering a few simple questions, you can discover a fasting schedule that seamlessly fits into your life.

Real-life Example: A good friend of my wife Sarah, a 42-year-old nurse with a rotating shift schedule. She found that a fixed eating window didn't suit her lifestyle. Instead, Sarah adjusts her 8-hour window based on her work shifts, ensuring she can eat a balanced meal before and after her shifts, demonstrating the 16/8 method's adaptability.

Reflection Section: *Document Your 16/8 Journey* Keep a daily log of your fasting hours, eating windows, how you feel physically and mentally, and any changes you notice. This reflection can help you fine-tune your fasting schedule to better suit your needs and preferences.

The 16/8 method stands out for its simplicity, flexibility, and the plethora of benefits it offers. Whether you're looking to manage your weight, improve metabolic health, or simply enhance your overall well-being, the 16/8 method provides a straightforward and adaptable approach to fasting that can fit into virtually any lifestyle. Remember, the key to success with intermittent fasting lies in finding a rhythm that feels natural and sustainable for you. With a bit of experimentation and patience, you can discover a fasting schedule that not only yields significant health benefits but also feels like a natural part of your daily routine.

2.2 Eat-Stop-Eat: The 24-Hour Reset

Imagine giving your digestive system a full day's break, allowing your body to focus on repair and rejuvenation. This is the essence of the Eat-Stop-Eat method, a fasting approach that involves a 24-hour fast once or twice a week. This method introduces a powerful pause in your weekly eating patterns, providing profound health benefits and offering a refreshingly straightforward way to improve your relationship with food.

Principles of Eat-Stop-Eat

The foundation of Eat-Stop-Eat is its simplicity: select one or two days a week where you abstain from eating for a full 24 hours. During this time, your body shifts into a state of fasting, tapping into stored fat for energy and initiating processes like autophagy, where cells clean out damaged components. The beauty of this method lies in its flexibility; you can decide which days to fast based on your schedule, making it adaptable to varying lifestyles.

How to Effectively Implement Eat-Stop-Eat

Initiating a 24-hour fast might seem daunting at first, but with a few strategic practices, it becomes more manageable:

- Choose Your Fasting Days Wisely: Opt for days when you're typically busier, as a packed schedule can help keep your mind off food.
- Hydrate Generously: Water, herbal teas, and black coffee are your allies during the fasting period, helping to curb hunger.
- Prepare Your Body: The day before fasting, eat balanced meals that are rich in fibre, protein, and healthy fats to keep you satiated longer.
- Ease Back into Eating: When breaking your fast, opt for a light meal that's easy to digest – think soups, salads, or smoothies – to gently awaken your digestive system.

Addressing Concerns with 24-Hour Fasting

It's natural to have reservations about this fasting method. Let's tackle a few common concerns:

- Maintaining Energy Levels: Surprisingly, many find their energy and focus increase during a 24-hour fast, thanks to the body's shift to fat-burning and reduced insulin levels.
- Managing Hunger: Hunger comes in waves and can often be quelled with hydration. When I felt hungry I would drink a pint

Chapter 2: Timing Over Tradition: The 16/8 Method Unpacked

of water, this always did the trick. Mindful distraction can also play a pivotal role – immerse yourself in activities that keep you engaged.

- Nutrient Deficiency: Since Eat-Stop-Eat is only once or twice a week, nutrient deficiencies are unlikely. Ensure your non-fasting days are filled with nutrient-dense foods to compensate. Also, my wife and I always made sure we took quality supplements

Personal Stories of Transformation

Hearing from those who've woven Eat-Stop-Eat into their lives illuminates the method's transformative potential:

- Mark's Journey: At 45, Mark felt his health slipping. Overweight and constantly tired, he sought a change. Eat-Stop-Eat not only helped him shed unwanted pounds but also instilled a newfound appreciation for the food he consumes, leading to healthier choices naturally.
- Linda's Experience: Linda, battling sugar cravings and afternoon slumps, found liberation through Eat-Stop-Eat. Her cravings diminished, her energy levels soared, and she discovered a sense of control over her eating habits she never thought possible.

Incorporating the Eat-Stop-Eat method into your life offers more than just physical health benefits; it fosters a deeper understanding of your body's cues and needs. It's a testament to the power of giving your body a rest, allowing it to reset and recharge. Though the idea of fasting for 24 hours may initially seem challenging, the adaptability of Eat-Stop-Eat means it can fit into almost any lifestyle, supporting long-term health and wellness without the need for drastic dietary changes.

2.3 The 5:2 Diet: Balancing Fasting and Eating

Diving straight into the heart of the 5:2 Diet reveals a method that redefines the art of fasting by harmonising days of normal eating with intervals of significantly reduced caloric intake. This approach, characterised by its 5 days of unrestricted eating followed by 2 days of consuming about 500-600 calories, marries the simplicity of intermittent fasting with the flexibility required by those of us steering through the complexities of mid-life responsibilities and health considerations.

The 5:2 Diet stands out for its unique blend of simplicity and effectiveness, making it particularly appealing for individuals seeking a less restrictive fasting regimen. On fasting days, caloric intake is limited to a quarter of an individual's regular intake, amounting to roughly 500 calories for women and 600 for men. These days are not consecutive, spreading the fasting periods out across the week to minimise the impact on energy levels and social life.

Health Advantages of the 5:2 Approach

- Weight Loss: Regular implementation of the 5:2 Diet can result in consistent weight loss, as the caloric deficit accrued on fasting days contributes to an overall reduction in weekly calorie intake.

- Metabolic Health: The intermittent nature of the 5:2 Diet can enhance metabolic flexibility, improving the body's ability to switch between burning carbohydrates and fats for energy, which is beneficial for weight management and metabolic health.

- Cognitive Function: Some evidence suggests that intermittent fasting regimens like the 5:2 Diet may bolster brain health, potentially reducing the risk of neurodegenerative diseases.

Creating a 5:2 Meal Plan

On fasting days, the goal is to maximise nutrient intake without exceeding the caloric limit, requiring a strategic approach to meal planning. Here are some tips for constructing a fasting day meal plan that is both satisfying and nutritionally rich:

Chapter 2: Timing Over Tradition: The 16/8 Method Unpacked

- Prioritise Protein: Lean protein sources like chicken breast, tofu, or fish can help keep you feeling full, all the while supporting muscle maintenance.
- Load Up on Vegetables: Low-calorie, high-fibre vegetables such as leafy greens, broccoli, and bell peppers can add volume and nutrients to meals without significantly impacting calorie count.
- Smart Use of Fats: Including small amounts of healthy fats from sources like avocados, nuts, or olive oil can enhance satiety and flavour.
- Stay Hydrated: Drinking plenty of water, herbal teas, or black coffee can help manage hunger pangs and maintain hydration.

Adapting the 5:2 Diet for Long-Term Success

For those embarking on the 5:2 journey, the initial weeks can be as much about mental adaptation as physical. Here are strategies to ensure this approach to intermittent fasting enriches your health over the long haul:

- Flexible Fasting Days: Choose fasting days that align with your schedule, opting for less hectic days when possible to ease the challenge of reduced caloric intake.
- Gradual Introduction: If jumping directly into two fasting days proves too challenging, start with one fasting day per week and gradually incorporate the second.
- Listen to Your Body: Pay close attention to how your body responds on fasting days. If you experience excessive fatigue or other adverse effects, consider adjusting the caloric limit slightly until you find a comfortable balance.
- Regular Reevaluation: As your body adapts and your health goals evolve, take time to reassess the effectiveness of the

5:2 Diet. Adjusting fasting calories or the distribution of macronutrients can help maintain progress and engagement.

Incorporating the 5:2 Diet into your lifestyle offers a pragmatic approach to intermittent fasting that respects the body's needs while challenging it to adapt and thrive. The beauty of this method lies in its blend of structure and flexibility, making it a viable option for those seeking a sustainable path to improved health and weight management. By focusing on nutrient-dense foods on fasting days and enjoying the freedom of traditional eating for the majority of the week, the 5:2 Diet presents a balanced approach to intermittent fasting that can be effortlessly woven into the fabric of everyday life.

2.4 Warrior Diet: Instinctive Eating with a Modern Twist

The Warrior Diet stands as a testament to the adaptability of intermittent fasting principles, taking inspiration from the ancient warrior societies who thrived on minimal daytime eating and feasting by night. This approach flips conventional eating patterns on their head, advocating for light consumption of raw fruits and vegetables during daylight hours and culminating in a substantial, nutrient-dense meal after sunset. This method, rooted in the instinctive eating habits of our ancestors, brings a refreshing simplicity to modern dietary practices.

The essence of the Warrior Diet lies in its flexibility and intuitive approach to nutrition, allowing for a deep connection with the body's natural hunger signals and nutritional needs. It encourages a period of under-eating during the day, where small servings of raw produce and minimal protein sources are consumed, thereby activating the body's survival instincts. As evening approaches, this diet transitions into a phase of overeating, where one substantial meal takes centre stage, providing a satisfying and nourishing end to the day.

Benefits of the Warrior Diet

Engaging with the Warrior Diet unfolds a variety of unique benefits, including:

Chapter 2: Timing Over Tradition: The 16/8 Method Unpacked

- Weight Loss and Body Composition: The structured under-eating and overeating phases can lead to a natural calorie deficit while preserving lean muscle mass, aiding in weight loss and improving body composition.

- Enhanced Energy Levels: Many find that light daytime eating enhances mental clarity and energy levels, possibly due to the body not being bogged down by heavy digestive processes.

- Improved Digestive Health: Eating one main meal a day gives the digestive system a prolonged break, potentially improving gut health and function.

- Flexibility and Simplicity: With its emphasis on instinctive eating, the Warrior Diet offers a liberating escape from the complexity of calorie counting and meticulous meal planning.

How to Implement the Warrior Diet

Transitioning to the Warrior Diet requires a mindful adjustment period, where listening to the body's cues becomes paramount. Here are steps to guide you through this transition:

1. Start with Light Daytime Nutrition: Gradually reduce your daytime food intake to small portions of raw fruits, vegetables, and lean proteins like nuts or yoghurt. This adjustment period helps accustom your body to the new eating pattern.

2. Stay Hydrated: Increase your water intake throughout the day to maintain hydration and help manage hunger.

3. Prepare for a Hearty Evening Meal: Plan a balanced, nutrient-rich meal for the evening, focusing on quality protein sources, whole grains, and plenty of vegetables to ensure all nutritional needs are met.

4. Pay Attention to Hunger Signals: Learn to distinguish between true hunger and habitual eating cues. The Warrior Diet

encourages eating in response to genuine hunger, not out of boredom or routine.

Customising the Warrior Diet

The true strength of the Warrior Diet lies in its adaptability to individual lifestyles and nutritional requirements. Here are suggestions for tailoring the diet to your personal needs:

- Adjust the Feasting Window: While the traditional approach recommends a single evening meal, some may find a slightly wider eating window more manageable. Adjusting this window to start earlier in the evening can accommodate family dinners or social engagements.

- Vary Daytime Intake According to Activity Levels: On days with higher physical activity, consider increasing your intake of protein and raw fruits during the day to support energy levels and recovery.

- Incorporate Nutrient Timing: Focus on consuming complex carbohydrates and proteins during your evening meal to aid in muscle repair and recovery overnight, especially if you engage in evening workouts.

- Experiment with Meal Composition: While the Warrior Diet emphasises a substantial evening meal, the composition of this meal can vary. Some may thrive on a higher protein intake, while others might find a focus on complex carbohydrates more satisfying. Experimenting with meal composition helps identify what best supports your energy levels and satiety.

Adopting the Warrior Diet is more than a change in eating habits; it's a shift towards a more instinctual relationship with food and nutrition. By tuning into the body's natural hunger signals and satisfying nutritional needs in a structured yet flexible manner, this diet not only supports physical health but also encourages a mindful, intuitive approach to eating. The Warrior Diet challenges modern dietary conventions,

Chapter 2: Timing Over Tradition: The 16/8 Method Unpacked

offering a path back to the basics of nutrition, where eating becomes a deliberate, nourishing act, rooted in the wisdom of our ancestors and tailored to the demands of contemporary life.

2.5 Time-Restricted Eating and Your Circadian Rhythm

Understanding the intricate dance between fasting and our biological clock unlocks a new dimension in achieving optimal health. The circadian rhythm, an internal process that regulates our sleep-wake cycle over roughly 24 hours, influences not just how we sleep but also how our body metabolises food. Synchronising eating times with this natural rhythm can lead to profound health improvements.

Linking Fasting to Your Biological Clock

The science behind circadian rhythms reveals that our bodies are designed to process nutrients more efficiently at certain times of the day. During daylight, our metabolism is more active, preparing us to consume and process food. As night falls, our body's focus shifts towards rest and repair, slowing down metabolic processes. Time-restricted eating leverages this knowledge, guiding us to eat in harmony with our body's natural states of activity and rest.

Benefits of Time-Restricted Eating

Adopting a time-restricted eating pattern, where one consumes all daily meals within a predetermined window, typically 8-10 hours, aligns with our circadian rhythm, offering several benefits:

- Enhanced Sleep Quality: Eating aligns with when our body is naturally more receptive to food, potentially improving sleep by preventing metabolic processes from interfering with rest.
- Boosted Energy Levels: Many report a notable increase in daytime energy, likely due to improved sleep quality and more efficient nutrient processing.
- Improved Metabolic Health: Time-restricted eating can lead to better blood sugar control, reduced risk of metabolic diseases,

and improved weight management, as it taps into our natural metabolic cycles.

Implementing Time-Restricted Eating

Starting a time-restricted eating regimen is straightforward, yet it requires mindful planning to ensure it complements your lifestyle:

1. Identify Your Ideal Eating Window: Begin by observing your daily routine to choose an 8-10 hour period for eating that feels natural. For most, a window that starts in the morning and ends in the evening works well.

2. Gradually Shorten Your Eating Window: If you're accustomed to eating over a longer span, reduce your window gradually. Start by cutting back an hour every few days until you reach your goal.

3. Plan Balanced Meals: To make the most of your eating window, include a mix of carbohydrates, proteins, and fats in your meals, focusing on whole foods to maximise nutrition.

4. Mindful Transitioning: Pay attention to how you feel as you adjust to your new eating schedule. It's normal to experience some hunger at first, but this typically diminishes as your body adapts.

Adapting to Lifestyle and Shifts in Circadian Rhythm

Our lives are dynamic, and so are our schedules. Here are tips for maintaining time-restricted eating amidst changes:

- Flexibility Is Key: If you know a late event is on the horizon, plan ahead by shifting your eating window that day to accommodate. A flexible approach ensures sustainability.

- Adjusting to Work Shifts: For those with irregular hours, like shift workers, aim to keep your eating window consistent with your active hours, even if they fall at night. Consistency helps your body adapt.

Chapter 2: Timing Over Tradition: The 16/8 Method Unpacked

- Listen and Adapt: As your routine changes, whether due to a new job or life stage, reassess your eating window. The goal is to find a pattern that feels right and supports your well-being.

Incorporating time-restricted eating into your life isn't about adhering to rigid rules but about finding a rhythm that aligns with your body's natural cycles. This approach not only simplifies the fasting process but also enhances its benefits, making it a practical and effective way to support your health. As you adjust your eating patterns, remember that the goal is to work with your body, not against it, fostering a harmonious balance that promotes overall well-being.

2.6 Personalising Your Fasting Plan: Listening to Your Body

Exploring the nuances of how our bodies react to different fasting schedules and food choices is pivotal in crafting a fasting plan that resonates with our unique physiological makeup. Recognizing and interpreting the signals our bodies send us—whether it's a growl in the stomach indicating hunger or a burst of energy signifying optimal fuel use—is the first step in fine-tuning our fasting approach.

Hunger cues and energy levels are just the tip of the iceberg when it comes to the body's means of communication. Changes in sleep quality, mood fluctuations, and even alterations in physical performance during workouts can all provide insights into how well a fasting regimen is serving us. For instance, feeling unusually fatigued or irritable may signal that your body is not getting the nutrients it needs within your current eating window, prompting a reassessment of your meal timing or composition.

With the myriad of fasting methods available, from the 16/8 method to more extended periods of fasting like the Eat-Stop-Eat approach, there exists a spectrum of options to experiment with. This experimentation is not about hopping from one method to another aimlessly but about finding the rhythm that aligns with your lifestyle, goals, and bodily responses. It might mean adjusting the length of your fasting window by an hour or two to see how it affects your energy levels or experimenting with different eating windows to better accommodate your social life or work schedule.

As we age, our bodies undergo significant changes that can influence how we respond to fasting. Metabolic rates, hormone levels, and activity patterns all evolve, necessitating adjustments to our fasting plans. A regimen that worked wonders in your forties might require tweaks to remain effective in your fifties and beyond. Regularly evaluating the impact of your fasting schedule on your health and adjusting it to align with your changing needs ensures that the benefits of fasting continue as you age.

Incorporating feedback from health professionals into your fasting plan is invaluable. Regular check-ups and consultations can provide a medical perspective on your fasting regimen, offering insights into how it's affecting aspects of your health that might not be immediately apparent, such as blood sugar levels, cholesterol, and blood pressure. This professional guidance can help you navigate the complexities of fasting with underlying health conditions, ensuring that your fasting approach is both safe and effective.

In sum, personalising your fasting plan is not a one-time task but an ongoing process of listening, experimenting, and adjusting. It's about building a dialogue with your body and responding to its needs with flexibility and mindfulness. By staying attuned to your body's signals, being open to trying different fasting methods, and adapting your approach as you age, you craft a fasting regimen that supports not just your physical health but your overall well-being. Consulting with healthcare professionals along the way ensures that your fasting journey is informed by a blend of personal insight and medical expertise.

As we wrap up this exploration of personalising your fasting plan, we're reminded of the broader journey we're on—a journey towards a healthier, more attuned life. The insights shared in this chapter pave the way for the discussions ahead, where we delve deeper into the

Chapter 2: Timing Over Tradition: The 16/8 Method Unpacked

practicalities of integrating fasting into our daily lives, ensuring that this powerful tool for health and wellness is wielded with knowledge, care, and respect.

Chapter 3: Setting the Stage for Success with Intermittent Fasting

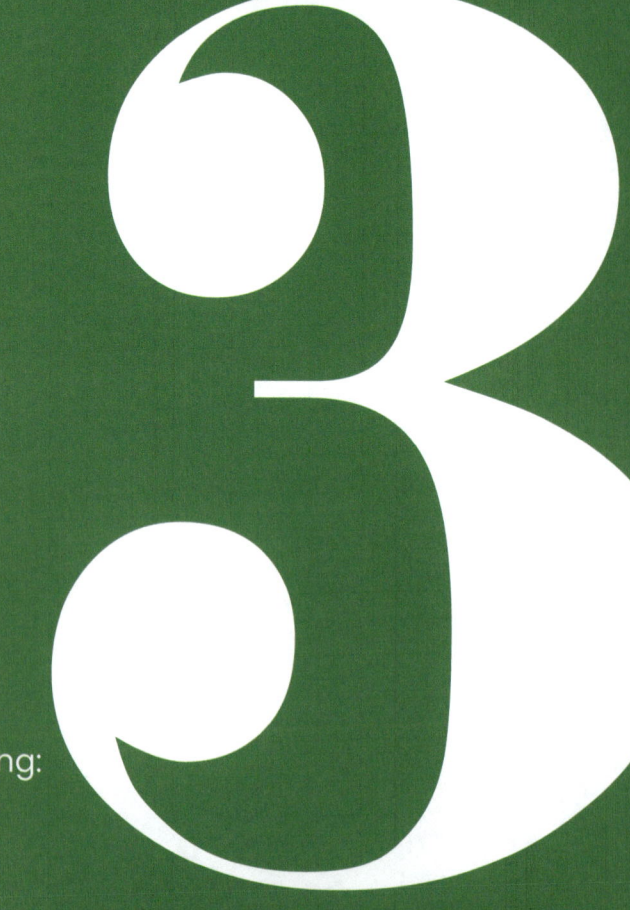

Chapter 3: Setting the Stage for Success with Intermittent Fasting

Stepping into the world of intermittent fasting is like tuning a musical instrument. The process requires attention, patience, and an understanding of the final sound you're aiming to achieve. Just as a well-tuned guitar creates harmony, a well-planned approach to fasting can harmonise your health, leading to a symphony of benefits. This chapter focuses on laying down the foundational strategies for a successful fasting experience, emphasising the importance of goal setting, managing expectations, and tracking progress.

Identifying Your WHY

The motivation behind why someone decides to start intermittent fasting varies widely. For some, it's about shedding extra pounds; for others, it's the allure of enhanced mental clarity or the desire to improve metabolic health. Pinpointing your motivation is crucial because it acts as your north star, guiding you through moments of doubt or when the initial excitement wanes. A clear understanding of your 'why' also helps in setting goals that are not just about the numbers on the scale but about enhancing your overall quality of life.

- Reflection Exercise: Take a moment to jot down all the reasons you're interested in intermittent fasting. Next to each reason, elaborate on how achieving this would make you feel and how it would impact your day-to-day life.

SMART Goals in Fasting

The concept of SMART goals isn't new, but its application to intermittent fasting can be a game-changer. Setting Specific, Measurable, Achievable, Relevant, and Time-bound goals ensures that your fasting plan is structured yet flexible enough to accommodate real life.

- Specific: Rather than a vague "I want to lose weight," aim for "I want to lose 10 pounds by incorporating the 16/8 intermittent fasting method into my daily routine."
- Measurable: Track your progress, be it through pounds lost,

improvement in energy levels, or better sleep quality.

- Achievable: Ensure your goal respects your current lifestyle. If you have a demanding job or family commitments, a fasting method requiring 24-hour fasts might not be the best starting point.
- Relevant: Your goal should align with your broader health objectives and your 'why'.
- Time-bound: Give yourself a realistic timeline to achieve your goal, keeping in mind that too tight a timeframe can lead to frustration.

Adjusting Expectations

It's easy to fall into the trap of expecting dramatic results instantly, especially with the numerous success stories circulating online. However, each body reacts differently to fasting. Some may see quick results, while others may find their progress more gradual. Adjusting your expectations to acknowledge that intermittent fasting is a marathon, not a sprint, can help maintain motivation over the long term. Importantly, progress in fasting isn't just measured by weight loss; improvements in energy levels, mental clarity, and a reduction in cravings are equally significant victories.

Tracking Progress Effectively

While stepping on the scale can provide some insight into your progress, it doesn't tell the whole story. Incorporating other methods to track your journey can offer a more comprehensive view of the benefits you're experiencing.

- Energy Levels: Keep a diary of how you feel during the day. Are you experiencing more stable energy levels, or are you still hitting that afternoon slump?
- Mental Clarity: Note any changes in your focus or cognitive function. Perhaps you're finding it easier to concentrate at work

Chapter 3: Setting the Stage for Success with Intermittent Fasting

or feeling more alert throughout the day.

- Fitness Improvements: If you exercise, track any changes in your performance or endurance. Sometimes, the progress is in being able to lift heavier, run longer, or simply feel more robust during your workouts.
- Visual Element: Progress Tracker Chart: Create a simple chart or use an app to log your daily fasting hours, mood, energy levels, and any other indicators of health you're focusing on. This visual representation of your journey can be a powerful motivator and a valuable tool for adjustments.

Setting the stage for success in intermittent fasting isn't just about choosing a method and starting; it's about aligning your goals with your motivations, setting realistic expectations, and tracking your progress in a way that captures the multifaceted benefits of fasting. Armed with these strategies, you're not just embarking on a dietary change but initiating a comprehensive lifestyle transformation that resonates with your individual needs and aspirations.

3.2 Kitchen Makeover: Preparing Your Space for Success

Creating an environment that supports your intermittent fasting goals is akin to setting the stage for a play where you are both the director and the lead actor. The kitchen, a central hub of nutrition and nourishment, requires special attention to ensure it aligns with your health aspirations. A well-organised and thoughtfully stocked kitchen can make the difference between a fasting plan that feels like an uphill battle and one that flows with ease.

Purging Processed Foods

Initiating this transformation begins with a purge of processed and unhealthy foods. This step is more than just clearing shelf space; it's about removing temptation and making a commitment to your health that's visible every time you open your pantry or fridge. Start by examining labels, and setting aside items high in added sugars, preservatives, and artificial ingredients. The goal isn't to waste, so consider donating unopened items to local food banks. This cleanses not only declutters your space but also your diet, paving the way for more mindful eating practices.

Stocking up on Fasting-Friendly Foods

With space cleared, the next step is to stock up on foods that nourish and satisfy. Focusing on whole, nutrient-dense options ensures that your eating windows provide the maximum benefit. Here's a quick list to consider:

- Fresh fruits and vegetables for hydration and fibre.
- Lean proteins like chicken, fish, and legumes for muscle repair and satiety.
- Healthy fats from avocados, nuts, and seeds support cell health and keep you feeling full longer.
- Whole grains for sustained energy and digestive health.
- Fermented foods such as yoghurt and kimchi support gut health.

Organisational Tips for a Fasting-Friendly Kitchen

Transforming your kitchen into a fasting-friendly zone also requires thoughtful organisation. Here are some tips to ensure healthy choices are always within easy reach:

- Dedicate sections of your fridge and pantry to fasting-approved snacks and ingredients, making them the first thing you see.
- Use clear containers for prepped fruits, veggies, and proteins, making it easier to grab a healthy option quickly.
- Keep a water pitcher front and centre in your fridge, perhaps infused with fruits or mint for a refreshing twist, encouraging hydration.

- Arrange your kitchen tools and gadgets in a way that supports your fasting lifestyle, like placing a blender on the counter for quick smoothies or protein shakes.

Mindful Grocery Shopping

Finally, adopting a mindful approach to grocery shopping can further reinforce your fasting goals. Before heading to the store, plan your meals and snacks for the week, considering the timing of your fasting windows. This plan helps avoid impulse buys and ensures you purchase only what supports your health objectives. While shopping, stick to the perimeter of the store where fresh produce, meats, and dairy are typically located. But, also venture into the aisles for whole grains, nuts, and seeds, being mindful to read labels and choose items with minimal added sugars and preservatives.

Incorporating these steps into your routine turns your kitchen into a bastion of support for your intermittent fasting journey. It ensures that every meal and snack consumed during your eating windows is chosen with intention, rich in nutrients, and aligned with your health goals. This environment not only facilitates adherence to your fasting schedule but also enriches your overall well-being, making your fasting experience as nourishing and effective as possible.

3.3 Understanding Hunger: Physical vs. Emotional

Navigating the waters of intermittent fasting introduces us to the complex interplay between physical hunger and emotional eating. Recognizing the nuances of these two types of hunger can significantly enhance your fasting experience, empowering you to respond to your body's needs more effectively.

Differentiating between physical and emotional hunger

Physical hunger, the body's natural response to needing fuel, develops gradually and can be satisfied with a variety of foods. It's often accompanied by clear physiological signals, such as a growling stomach or a slight dip in energy levels. Emotional hunger, on the other hand, arises suddenly and craves specific comfort foods. It's driven by feelings rather than actual energy needs and tends to lead to mindless eating that doesn't satisfy the emotional void it aims to fill.

- Physical hunger signals: Gradual onset, open to different foods, satisfied once full.
- Emotional hunger cues: Sudden craving, specific food focus, often followed by guilt or dissatisfaction.

Coping strategies for emotional eating

When the urge to eat is driven by emotions rather than physical hunger, finding strategies to address the root cause is key. Here are several approaches to managing emotional cravings without derailing your fasting plan:

- Pause and reflect: Before reaching for food, take a moment to assess the true nature of your hunger. Are you eating out of boredom, stress, or loneliness?
- Find alternative outlets: If you identify an emotional trigger, seek out non-food-related activities to address that emotion. A brisk walk, a chat with a friend, or engaging in a hobby can provide the distraction or comfort you seek.
- Create a comfort list: Compile a list of activities that bring you joy and comfort that aren't food-related. Having this list ready can provide quick alternatives when emotional hunger strikes.

The role of mindfulness in managing hunger

Mindfulness, the practice of being fully present and engaged at the moment, can be a powerful tool in distinguishing between types of hunger and responding appropriately. By tuning into your body's signals and eating with intention, you can better understand your hunger cues and make choices that align with your body's needs.

- Mindful eating practices: During your eating windows, focus on the sensory experience of eating—savour each bite, notice the

- Body scan meditation: Regularly practising body scans can heighten your awareness of physical sensations, including hunger, helping you to distinguish them from emotional signals more effectively.

Reframing hunger as part of the fasting experience

Viewing hunger as an enemy to be battled can make fasting a stressful experience. Instead, consider reframing hunger as a natural and expected part of the fasting process. This shift in perspective recognizes hunger as a signal that your body is tapping into its fat stores for energy, a positive step towards your health goals. It's also an opportunity to strengthen your willpower and deepen your understanding of your body's cues.

- Anticipate and plan for hunger: Knowing that hunger will come allows you to prepare mentally and have strategies in place to manage it, such as staying hydrated, keeping busy, or using mindfulness techniques.
- Embrace the benefits: Remind yourself of the reasons behind your fasting choice and the benefits you're aiming to achieve. This can help transform hunger from a challenge into a marker of progress.

Incorporating these strategies into your intermittent fasting plan enables a more nuanced understanding of hunger, equipping you with the tools to navigate both physical and emotional cravings. By doing so, you honour your body's natural rhythms and needs, fostering a healthier relationship with food and with yourself.

3.4 The Importance of Hydration

In the realm of intermittent fasting, the spotlight often shines brightest on what and when we eat. Yet, there's another player in this performance that deserves equal billing: hydration. The role of staying hydrated, particularly during fasting periods, is pivotal for ensuring the body operates at peak efficiency. It's like oil in an engine, keeping everything running smoothly and preventing the gears from grinding to a halt.

Hydration's Role in Fasting

During fasting windows, the body shifts its energy sourcing, tapping into stored fat for fuel. This metabolic switcheroo, while beneficial for weight loss and health, also triggers increased needs for fluid as the body processes and eliminates byproducts of fat breakdown. Moreover, without regular food intake, which typically accounts for a portion of our daily fluid intake, the risk of dehydration subtly inches upward. Adequate hydration supports not only metabolic processes but also brain function, keeping focus sharp and mood stable. It's the silent partner in the fasting equation, ensuring that the absence of food doesn't lead to a deficit in body function.

Best Fluids for Staying Hydrated

While water is the undefeated champion of hydration, it's not the only contender. During fasting periods, the goal is to consume fluids that maintain hydration without breaking the fast. Here's where variety comes into play:

- Water: The cornerstone of hydration, plain water is always a perfect choice. It's the zero-calorie, zero-complication way to stay hydrated.

- Herbal teas: Offering a bouquet of flavours, herbal teas can make hydration a sensory pleasure. Whether it's the calming notes of chamomile or the zesty kick of ginger, herbal teas add variety without adding calories.

- Black coffee: For many, the ritual of morning coffee is non-negotiable. Thankfully, black coffee, sans sugar or cream, is fasting-friendly. Its diuretic effect is minimal for those accustomed to caffeine, making it a viable option for hydration.

Chapter 3: Setting the Stage for Success with Intermittent Fasting

Recognizing Signs of Dehydration

Staying vigilant for dehydration's telltale signs ensures that fasting doesn't compromise hydration. These indicators act as the body's SOS, signalling it's time to up the fluid intake:

- Fatigue: An unexpected wave of tiredness during a fast might not just be hunger; it could be dehydration.
- Headaches: A common distress signal from the body, a headache during fasting might be the brain's way of asking for more fluids.
- Dry mouth or thirst: While this seems obvious, it's often overlooked. If you're feeling parched, you're already on the path to dehydration.
- Dark urine: The colour of your urine is a direct line to your hydration status. Aim for a light straw colour as a sign of good hydration.

Tips for Incorporating More Fluids into Your Day

Integrating more fluids into your fasting routine doesn't have to feel like a chore. With a bit of creativity and planning, you can ensure you're meeting your hydration needs without constant reminders to "drink more water."

- Start your day with a glass of water: Making this first act in the morning sets a positive tone for hydration throughout the day.
- Keep a water bottle handy: A visible, easily accessible water bottle acts as a constant reminder to take sips throughout the day.
- Set reminders: In our busy lives, it's easy to forget to hydrate. Setting periodic reminders on your phone or computer can keep hydration on your radar.
- Spice up your water: Adding slices of lemon, cucumber, or berries to your water can make reaching for that glass more appealing.

- Embrace herbal teas: Explore the wide world of herbal teas as a way to hydrate with flavour and warmth, adding a comforting ritual to your fasting window.

Incorporating these hydration strategies into your intermittent fasting plan ensures that your body remains well-oiled and functioning optimally, supporting your health goals without the added complication of dehydration. Remember, while fasting focuses on when and what you eat, never underestimate the power of staying hydrated. It's the silent backbone of your fasting regimen, supporting every step of your health journey with the simplicity and efficacy of a well-timed sip of water.

3.5 Supplements and Intermittent Fasting: What You Need to Know

When exploring the synergy between intermittent fasting, nutrition, and wellness, the topic of supplements naturally arises. In this fasting landscape, understanding how to effectively incorporate supplements can optimise health benefits while ensuring the fast remains effective.

Navigating Supplementation While Fasting

The first step is distinguishing which supplements are fasting-friendly and which might inadvertently break your fast. Generally, most vitamin and mineral supplements can be taken without disrupting the fasting state, particularly if they are calorie-free and do not stimulate insulin production. However, some supplements, especially those in gummy form or containing added sugars, could potentially interrupt the fasting process. Key supplements often recommended include:

- Multivitamins: To fill any nutritional gaps that might occur, especially during the initial adjustment period to fasting.
- Electrolytes: Essential during longer fasting periods to maintain hydration and prevent electrolyte imbalances.
- Omega-3 fatty acids: Beneficial for heart health and inflammation, usually fine to take while fasting as they do not contain calories that can break a fast.

Chapter 3: Setting the Stage for Success with Intermittent Fasting

Essential Nutrients During Fasting Windows

Focusing on key nutrients during eating windows ensures the body receives the support it needs to thrive under a fasting regimen. These essential nutrients include:

- Protein: Critical for muscle repair and growth, aim to consume adequate amounts of protein during your eating windows.
- Fibre: Found in fruits, vegetables, and whole grains, fibre supports digestive health and can enhance the feeling of fullness.
- Calcium and Vitamin D: Important for bone health, these can be sourced from dairy products or fortified alternatives.
- Iron: Especially important for women and those on plant-based diets, iron supports blood health and energy levels.

Balancing these nutrients during eating windows not only supports overall health but also prepares the body for the next fasting period, ensuring it has the resources needed for cellular repair and energy production.

Timing Supplements With Your Fasting Schedule

To maximise the effectiveness of supplements and avoid breaking your fast, consider the timing of your supplement intake. Water-soluble vitamins (such as B vitamins and vitamin C) and electrolytes can often be taken during fasting periods as they do not require food for absorption and are unlikely to break a fast. Fat-soluble vitamins (such as vitamins A, D, E, and K), however, are best taken with meals to enhance absorption. Here's a quick guide:

- Morning (Fasting Period): Electrolytes, water-soluble vitamins.
- During Eating Windows: Multivitamins, omega-3 fatty acids, fat-soluble vitamins, protein supplements.
- Evening (If Eating Window is Closed): Fibre supplements (if needed) with a glass of water.

This timing ensures your body receives nutrients when they can be most effectively absorbed and utilised, supporting your fasting and health goals.

Consulting with Healthcare Providers

Before adding any supplements to your routine, a conversation with a healthcare provider is invaluable. They can offer personalised advice based on your health history, current medications, and specific dietary needs. This is particularly important for those managing chronic conditions or taking prescribed medications, as certain supplements can interact with medications or may not be recommended based on individual health issues. A healthcare provider can also suggest blood tests to identify any nutrient deficiencies, ensuring that your supplement choices are informed and targeted to your needs.

In navigating the world of supplements alongside intermittent fasting, the focus remains on supporting your body's health and fasting goals. By choosing the right supplements, timing their intake thoughtfully, and seeking professional guidance, you can enhance the benefits of intermittent fasting and ensure your body receives the nutritional support it needs. This careful approach to supplementation enriches the fasting experience, empowering you with the knowledge and strategies to support your health journey.

3.6 Building a Support System

Navigating the waves of intermittent fasting can sometimes feel like sailing in uncharted waters. Having a crew of supporters and fellow navigators can make all the difference in weathering the storms and celebrating the sunny days. A robust support system not only fuels your motivation but also provides a lifeline during those moments when your resolve might waver.

Chapter 3: Setting the Stage for Success with Intermittent Fasting

Finding Fasting Buddies

Creating connections with others who are also navigating the intermittent fasting landscape can significantly enrich your experience. Here are a few ways to find your fasting crew:

- Local wellness groups: Check community boards or social media for local groups focused on health, wellness, and nutrition. Many cities have meet-up groups centred around these themes.
- Gym or fitness class connections: Strike up conversations about nutrition and fasting with workout buddies. You might find others who are curious or already practising intermittent fasting.
- Workplace wellness networks: Many workplaces have health and wellness programs or interest groups. Joining these can be a great way to find support among colleagues.

Leveraging Online Communities and Resources

The digital age brings the world to our fingertips, including a wealth of online communities and resources dedicated to intermittent fasting. Here's where to look:

- Social media groups: Platforms like Facebook and Reddit host numerous intermittent fasting groups where members share experiences, challenges, and successes.
- Blogs and forums: Websites dedicated to intermittent fasting often have comment sections, forums, or guest post opportunities where you can connect with like-minded individuals.
- Mobile apps: Many intermittent fasting apps offer community features, allowing you to join challenges, share progress, and exchange tips with other users.

Communicating Your Fasting Goals with Friends and Family

While finding support among those who share your intermittent fasting goals is invaluable, bringing friends and family into your support circle is equally important. Here's how to approach the conversation:

- Share your 'why': Explain the reasons behind your choice to practise intermittent fasting, focusing on the health benefits and personal goals you aim to achieve.
- Clarify what support looks like to you: Whether it's not offering you snacks outside your eating window or simply being a listening ear, let them know how they can best support you.
- Educate with kindness: There might be misconceptions or concerns about intermittent fasting. Sharing articles, videos, or personal testimonials can help alleviate worries and foster understanding.
- Invite participation: While not everyone will want to join you in fasting, inviting them to share a meal during your eating window can be a way to include them in your new routine.

Fostering a support system as you navigate intermittent fasting adds a layer of richness to the experience. It transforms the journey from a solitary endeavour to a shared adventure, filled with encouragement, learning, and mutual growth. Whether finding allies among peers, connecting with a global online community, or inviting friends and family to understand and support your goals, the strength of your support network can be a pivotal factor in the success and enjoyment of your intermittent fasting journey.

Now, as we close this chapter, remember that intermittent fasting is not just about the hours you eat and fast; it's about integrating this practice into a life filled with relationships, activities, and goals. The support you cultivate, both near and far, plays a crucial role in this integration. It's about more than just shared experiences or advice on overcoming challenges; it's about building connections that nourish

Chapter 3: Setting the Stage for Success with Intermittent Fasting

you as much as the food you choose to eat during your feeding windows.

As we move forward, let's keep in mind the importance of community, communication, and support in enriching our fasting experience and achieving our health and wellness goals.

Chapter 4: Night and Day: Syncing Fasting with Life's Rhythms

Chapter 4: Night and Day: Syncing Fasting with Life's Rhythms

In the dance of day and night, there's a rhythm that guides not just the natural world but also our internal clocks. It's in the ebb and flow of these cycles that we find the keys to unlocking a more harmonious relationship with food, sleep, and ultimately, our health. This chapter shines a light on an often-overlooked ally in our quest for wellness: sleep. We'll explore how this silent partner works hand in hand with intermittent fasting, offering strategies to enhance rest, align eating windows with our body's natural rhythms, and address the sleep disturbances that can sometimes accompany a fasting lifestyle.

Sleep: The Unsung Hero of Weight Loss

The connection between sleep and weight management is more profound than most realise. Good quality sleep acts as a foundation for effective weight loss and overall health, especially when combined with intermittent fasting. During restful sleep, our bodies undergo repair and rejuvenation, processes that are critical for metabolism, muscle growth, and hormone balance. These overnight activities help regulate hunger hormones like ghrelin and leptin, making it easier to adhere to fasting periods without succumbing to cravings. It's during deep sleep that the body also burns fat more efficiently, thanks to an increased metabolic rate.

Tips for Improving Sleep While Fasting

Creating an environment conducive to restful sleep can significantly enhance the effectiveness of intermittent fasting. Consider these strategies for better sleep:

- Optimise your sleeping environment: Ensure your bedroom is cool, dark, and quiet. Consider blackout curtains, white noise machines, or earplugs to block out disturbances.
- Establish a pre-sleep routine: Engage in calming activities like reading or taking a warm bath to signal to your body that it's time to wind down. Avoid screens at least an hour before bed to minimise blue light exposure, which can disrupt sleep cycles.

- Mind your caffeine intake: Limit caffeine consumption to the early part of your eating window to prevent it from affecting your sleep.

The Impact of Eating Windows on Sleep

The timing of your fasting and eating windows can profoundly affect your sleep quality. Eating too close to bedtime, especially large meals, can lead to discomfort and disruptions in sleep. On the other hand, finishing your last meal a few hours before sleep can improve sleep quality by allowing your digestive system to rest. For those practising time-restricted eating, aligning your eating window to end at least 2-3 hours before your usual bedtime supports natural sleep patterns and enhances overnight metabolic processes.

Dealing with Sleep Disturbances During Fasting

For some, the initial transition to intermittent fasting can bring about changes in sleep patterns. Here are ways to navigate these challenges:

- Stay hydrated during your eating window: Dehydration can lead to sleep disturbances. Ensuring adequate fluid intake can prevent waking up thirsty in the middle of the night.
- Balance your meals: Include a mix of protein, healthy fats, and complex carbohydrates in your last meal to promote satiety and stabilise blood sugar levels through the night.
- Consider light exercise: Gentle activities like yoga or stretching in the evening can promote relaxation and improve sleep quality.

Visual Element: Infographic on 'Building the Perfect Pre-Sleep Routine' This infographic provides a step-by-step guide to creating a calming pre-sleep routine, including ideal room temperatures, recommended calming activities, and tips for minimising electronic usage before bed.

Chapter 4: Night and Day: Syncing Fasting with Life's Rhythms

Interactive Element: Sleep Quality and Fasting Log Keep track of your sleep quality alongside your fasting schedule in a log. Note any changes in how easily you fall asleep, the number of times you wake up during the night, and how rested you feel in the morning. Over time, you may notice patterns that can help you adjust your fasting and eating windows for better sleep.

Textual Element: Case Study on Eating Windows and Sleep Explore real-life scenarios where individuals adjusted their eating windows and implemented sleep-enhancing practices, resulting in improved sleep quality and more effective fasting outcomes. These case studies highlight the adjustments made, the challenges faced, and the strategies that led to success.

In this exploration of sleep and intermittent fasting, we uncover the intricate relationship between rest and metabolism. By prioritising sleep as a crucial component of your fasting plan, you not only support your body's natural rhythms but also enhance the effectiveness of your fasting efforts. The strategies shared here aim to guide you in creating a fasting schedule that not only respects your dietary goals but also nurtures your body's need for rest and rejuvenation.

4.2 Exercise and Intermittent Fasting: Finding the Right Balance

Marrying exercise with intermittent fasting paints a vivid picture of enhanced health benefits, drawing from each practice's strengths to foster a synergistic effect on fat loss, muscle gain, and overall vitality. This section unwraps the layers of integrating physical activity into your fasting lifestyle, offering insights into the types of exercises that align with fasting states and strategies for timing workouts for maximal benefit. It also underscores the importance of tuning into your body's signals to tailor exercise intensity, ensuring a harmonious balance between fasting and fitness.

The Synergy of Exercise and Fasting

The fusion of fasting and exercise ignites a powerful metabolic shift, accelerating fat burning while preserving muscle mass. Fasting states prime the body to tap into fat stores for energy, a process that exercise intensifies, leading to more significant fat loss. Concurrently, exercising during fasting periods, especially resistance training, sends signals to preserve muscle, even in a calorie deficit. This dual approach not only shapes the body but also enhances metabolic flexibility, teaching it to efficiently switch between energy sources.

Tailored Exercise Recommendations During Fasting

Choosing the right type of exercise during fasting hinges on understanding how different activities interact with the body's current energy state. Here are two pillars of exercise that complement fasting:

- Strength Training: Lifting weights or engaging in bodyweight exercises during fasting windows can enhance growth hormone release, crucial for muscle preservation and growth. Since these activities primarily use glycogen stores, they're effective even when energy intake is low.
- Low-Intensity Cardio: Activities like walking, cycling, or swimming at low intensity are perfectly suited for fasting periods. They burn fat directly as fuel, capitalising on the body's fasting state, and are gentle enough to prevent muscle catabolism.

Orchestrating Workout Timing with Fasting

To fully harness the benefits of combining exercise with intermittent fasting, the timing of workouts is key. Here's how to align your exercise routine with your fasting schedule:

- Strength Training: For those following a daily fast, such as the 16/8 method, scheduling strength workouts towards the end of the fasting period and before the first meal can optimise

Chapter 4: Night and Day: Syncing Fasting with Life's Rhythms

muscle preservation and fat loss. This timing takes advantage of the natural spike in growth hormone levels that fasting induces.

- Low-Intensity Cardio: This can be flexibly performed at any point during the fasting window, as it gently utilises fat stores without overly taxing the body. Morning hours are ideal for many, infusing the day with energy without compromising the fasting state.

Heeding Your Body's Cues

While the integration of exercise into fasting brings undeniable benefits, it also demands a heightened awareness of your body's feedback. Here are considerations to ensure this combination supports rather than depletes your health:

- Monitor Energy Levels: Some days, your energy may not peak as usual, signalling the need to dial back exercise intensity or duration. Respecting these cues ensures you're supporting your body without overextension.

- Watch for Recovery Signs: Adequate recovery, signalled by the absence of prolonged soreness or fatigue, indicates your exercise routine aligns well with your fasting schedule. Persistent fatigue or reduced performance might mean it's time to adjust either your workout intensity, fasting duration, or nutrient intake during eating windows.

- Stay Flexible: Your body's response to fasting and exercise will evolve. What works well one month may need adjustment the next. This fluid approach allows you to continuously refine your routine in response to your body's changing needs.

In weaving exercise into the fabric of intermittent fasting, we embrace a strategy that amplifies the benefits of both practices. This dynamic pairing not only accelerates physical transformation but also enhances metabolic health and energy levels. By selecting suitable exercises, strategically timing workouts, and remaining attuned to the

4.3 Managing Stress to Enhance the Benefits of Fasting

In the intricate dance of well-being, stress often steps on the toes of our best intentions, particularly when navigating the waters of intermittent fasting. The way stress influences our fasting journey is multifaceted, intertwining with our hormone levels and eating behaviours, potentially muddying the waters of our progress. Recognizing stress as a significant factor allows us to not only address its impact but also harness fasting's role in building a more resilient response to stress. Here, we explore practical stress reduction techniques, understand fasting's contribution to stress resilience, and construct a tailored plan to manage stress, ensuring it supports rather than hinders our fasting efforts.

Stress's Impact on Fasting and Health

When stress enters the picture, it doesn't do so quietly. It brings along cortisol, a hormone that, at elevated levels, can upset our metabolic balance. This disruption can lead to cravings for sugary or fatty foods, making adherence to fasting windows more challenging. Additionally, stress can trigger emotional eating, a behaviour that often leads to consuming food for comfort rather than nourishment, creating a cycle that can be hard to break. Recognizing these patterns is the first step in creating a buffer against stress's impact on our fasting and overall health.

Stress Reduction Techniques

A toolkit of stress reduction strategies can be a lifeline on your fasting journey. Incorporating these practices can not only alleviate stress but also enhance the clarity and focus needed to maintain your fasting schedule:

- Meditation: A few minutes of meditation daily can significantly lower stress levels. Whether it's guided imagery, mindfulness

Chapter 4: Night and Day: Syncing Fasting with Life's Rhythms

meditation, or simply focusing on your breath, the key is consistency.

- Deep Breathing Exercises: The 4-7-8 technique, wherein you breathe in for 4 seconds, hold for 7 seconds, and exhale for 8 seconds, can be a quick and effective method to reduce stress anytime, anywhere.
- Yoga: Beyond its physical benefits, yoga offers a mental reprieve from stress, with certain poses particularly effective in fostering relaxation and mental calm.
- Nature Walks: Time spent in nature can decrease stress hormones and enhance mood. Even a brief walk can shift your perspective and reduce stress. Personally, this is my go-to stress relief. Being in nature, especially among the trees, connects us to our natural tempo-rhythm. I come up with all my best ideas in the woods.

Incorporating these techniques into your routine doesn't require large chunks of time; even short intervals can be profoundly beneficial. The key is making them a regular part of your day, creating moments of calm amidst the hustle.

The Role of Fasting in Stress Resilience

Fasting, by its nature, teaches the body and mind discipline, creating a framework within which we learn to handle discomfort, like hunger or stress, with grace. Over time, this discipline fosters resilience, equipping us to face stress with a steadier hand. Interestingly, fasting can also physiologically bolster our resilience to stress. By improving metabolic health, enhancing brain function, and reducing inflammation, fasting strengthens our internal systems, making them more adept at managing stress's biochemical impacts.

Creating a Stress-Management Plan

A personalised plan to manage stress, particularly in the context of fasting, can be a cornerstone of your wellness strategy. Crafting this plan involves a few key components:

- Identify Stress Triggers: Keep a journal for a week or two, noting when stress levels rise. Look for patterns. Is it work, family, health, or perhaps the fasting itself that spikes stress?
- Choose Your Techniques: Based on your triggers and what resonates with you, select a few stress reduction techniques to focus on. If meditation doesn't suit you, perhaps deep breathing or yoga might.
- Schedule Time for Stress Reduction: Incorporate your chosen techniques into your daily schedule as non-negotiable appointments with yourself. Even 5-10 minutes can make a difference.
- Monitor and Adjust: Regularly assess the effectiveness of your stress management plan. What's working? What isn't? Adjust your techniques and their frequency as needed to find what best supports your needs.

This proactive approach to managing stress ensures that your fasting journey is not only about the food you eat or don't eat but also about nurturing a mindset that supports lasting well-being. Through meditation, deep breathing, yoga, or simply spending time in nature, you can build a foundation that not only withstands stress but also enhances the profound benefits of intermittent fasting. With a tailored stress management plan in hand, you're equipped to navigate the challenges of fasting and life with resilience, paving the way for a healthier, more balanced existence.

4.4 Mindful Eating: Enhancing Your Relationship with Food

In the realm of intermittent fasting, where the clock dictates the ebb and flow of our eating patterns, there lies an opportunity not just to reconsider what we eat, but how we eat it. This section introduces mindful eating, a practice that transforms mealtime from a routine task into a deliberate act of nourishment and gratitude. Mindful eating isn't a diet but a way of eating that encourages a deep connection with food, heightening the experience of each bite and aligning it with the body's true needs.

Principles of Mindful Eating

At its core, mindful eating is about engaging fully with the act of eating, using all senses to enjoy food and becoming aware of the mind and body's cues. It's a practice rooted in mindfulness, the art of being present and fully engaged with whatever we're doing at the moment without judgement. When applied to eating, it asks us to slow down, pay attention to the taste, texture, and aroma of our food, and notice the effects food has on our feelings and body. This awareness can transform the eating experience, turning it into a source of pleasure and satisfaction rather than just a means to an end.

Benefits of Mindful Eating in Intermittent Fasting

Integrating mindful eating into your fasting routine offers numerous benefits that can enhance the fasting experience:

- Improves Satiety: By slowing down and savouring each bite, you give your body time to recognize fullness, often leading to eating less while feeling more satisfied.
- Enhances Food Enjoyment: Taking the time to truly taste and enjoy your food can make meals more satisfying, helping to eliminate feelings of deprivation during fasting periods.
- Reduces Cravings: Mindful eating helps in distinguishing between true hunger and emotional or boredom-driven cravings, aiding in making healthier food choices.

- Encourages Nutritional Choices: With a focus on the experience of eating, there's a natural gravitation towards foods that offer deeper satisfaction and nourishment, supporting overall health.

Practices for Mindful Eating

Incorporating mindful eating into your routine doesn't require sweeping changes but rather a shift in attention. Here are practical ways to start:

- Eat Slowly: Take time to chew your food thoroughly, allowing yourself to fully experience the flavours and textures.
- Limit Distractions: Turn off the TV, put away your phone, and make mealtime an opportunity to disconnect from the outside world and connect with your food.
- Engage All Senses: Before eating, take a moment to appreciate the appearance and aroma of your food. As you eat, pay attention to the taste and texture.
- Listen to Your Body: Tune into your body's hunger and fullness cues. Start eating when you're truly hungry and stop when you're comfortably full, even if there's food left on your plate.

Overcoming Mindless Eating Habits

For many, eating can become an automatic behaviour, something we do while distracted, stressed, or bored. To shift away from mindless eating and embrace mindfulness, consider these strategies:

- Identify Triggers: Keep a food journal to note when and why you eat. Do you reach for snacks when stressed or bored? Recognizing these patterns is the first step in changing them.
- Create New Routines: If you find you eat mindlessly in certain situations (like watching TV), create new routines that don't involve food, such as knitting or doodling.
- Practice Gratitude: Before eating, take a moment to express gratitude for your food and consider the journey it took to reach

Chapter 4: Night and Day: Syncing Fasting with Life's Rhythms

your plate. This can create a moment of pause and reflection that fosters mindful eating.

- Mindful Snacking: If you snack, put a serving on a plate instead of eating from the package. Sit down and eat it slowly, savouring each bite, to transform snacking into a mindful practice.

In wrapping up, mindful eating stands as a beacon in the intermittent fasting landscape, guiding us towards a deeper connection with our food and ourselves. It teaches us to eat with intention and attention, transforming mealtime into a pleasurable, nourishing experience that supports our fasting goals. By slowing down, savouring each bite, and tuning into our body's cues, we open the door to a more mindful, healthful approach to eating that can enrich our lives far beyond the fasting window.

4.5 Navigating Social Events and Holidays

In the tapestry of life, social gatherings and holidays are vibrant threads, weaving joy and connection into our daily existence. Yet, for those of us integrating intermittent fasting into our lives, these occasions can present unique challenges, testing our resolve and flexibility. The key to maintaining your fasting schedule without missing out on the richness of shared meals and celebrations lies in preparation, communication, and mindful choices.

Mastering Social Eating and Fasting

The art of balancing social engagements with fasting is akin to walking a tightrope, requiring focus and a strategy to maintain equilibrium. Here are several tactics to navigate this path with ease:

- Plan Ahead: Familiarise yourself with the event's timing and menu. If it falls outside your eating window, consider adjusting your fasting schedule for the day. A slight shift can allow you to partake in the festivities without breaking your fasting commitments.

- Bring a Fasting-Friendly Dish: When attending potlucks or family dinners, contribute a dish that aligns with your dietary preferences. This ensures you'll have at least one item you can enjoy without compromising your fasting goals.
- Focus on Hydration: Keep a glass of water or a fasting-approved beverage in hand throughout the event. It helps manage hunger and keeps your hands and mouth occupied, making it easier to engage in conversations without gravitating toward unplanned snacking.

Communicating Your Needs to Hosts

Approaching conversations about your fasting lifestyle with grace and gratitude can foster understanding and support from those around you. Here's how you might approach this dialogue:

- Share Your Approach: In casual conversations, express your enthusiasm for the positive changes you're experiencing with intermittent fasting. Framing it as a personal wellness experiment can pique interest and garner support.
- Be Specific About Your Needs: If a close friend or family member is hosting, they might appreciate knowing how they can support you. Suggest simple adjustments, like scheduling the meal within your eating window, that can make a big difference for you.
- Express Gratitude: Always thank your hosts for their understanding and flexibility. Acknowledging their efforts to accommodate your needs strengthens relationships and makes future gatherings easier to navigate.

Making Wise Choices at Social Events

Armed with a plan and clear communication, making healthy choices at social gatherings becomes more intuitive. Keep these tips in mind:

Chapter 4: Night and Day: Syncing Fasting with Life's Rhythms

- Prioritise Protein and Vegetables: When faced with a buffet or dinner table, fill your plate first with proteins and vegetables. These nutrient-dense foods offer satiety and align well with most fasting regimens.
- Practice Portion Control: With tempting dishes in abundance, decide in advance to sample in moderation. Small servings allow you to taste without overindulging, keeping you within the bounds of your dietary goals.
- Mindful Eating: Even in a social setting, take the time to savour each bite. Eating slowly and with intention enhances the enjoyment of your meal and helps prevent overeating.

Balancing Enjoyment and Goals

Finding joy in social occasions while staying true to your fasting goals is entirely achievable with the right mindset. Here's how to strike that balance:

- Flexibility Is Your Friend: Remember that intermittent fasting is part of a larger lifestyle aimed at improving your health and happiness. Occasional adjustments to your fasting schedule to accommodate special events are not only acceptable but necessary for a balanced life.
- Savour the Moment: Place emphasis on the company and conversation, rather than the food alone. The memories made with loved ones are far more nourishing than any meal.
- Reflect on Your Experience: After the event, take a moment to reflect on what went well and what you might adjust next time. This continuous learning process will refine your approach to social eating, making each occasion more enjoyable and less stressful.

In navigating the social aspects of intermittent fasting, we discover that our dietary choices do not have to isolate us from cherished traditions and gatherings. Instead, with thoughtful planning, open communication, and mindful choices, we can fully engage in the joy of social events and holidays while honouring our commitment to health and well-being. This balanced approach ensures that our fasting journey enriches our lives, deepening connections with others while nurturing our physical and emotional health.

4.6 Intermittent Fasting While Travelling

Navigating the intricacies of intermittent fasting becomes a unique puzzle when the backdrop changes from the familiar settings of home and work to the unpredictable environments encountered while travelling. Whether it's a business trip, a family vacation, or a solo adventure, maintaining a fasting routine on the road introduces a new set of challenges, from time zone shifts to meal planning in unfamiliar territories.

Facing the Challenges on the Road

Travel, by its nature, disrupts our routines, making the adherence to a fasting schedule more complex. Airports, with their limited healthy food options, long flights that span meal times, and the social aspect of dining out in new places, all pose potential hurdles. Additionally, the excitement and stress of travel can trigger changes in appetite and eating patterns, making it tempting to stray from fasting disciplines.

Strategizing Ahead for Travel

With a bit of foresight, these challenges become manageable. Planning is pivotal:

- Research your destination: Look for restaurants and grocery stores that offer healthy, fasting-friendly options. Many places now cater to various dietary preferences, making it easier to find meals that fit your eating window and nutritional needs.
- Pack smart: Bring along non-perishable, fasting-friendly snacks and meals. Nuts, seeds, protein bars (low in sugar), and even

Chapter 4: Night and Day: Syncing Fasting with Life's Rhythms

pre-packed salads can be lifesavers during travel.

- Stay hydrated: Carry a refillable water bottle to ensure you stay hydrated, especially crucial during flights where the temptation to snack can often be a misinterpreted signal of dehydration.

Choosing Fasting-Friendly Snacks and Meals

What you eat while travelling can significantly impact how well you maintain your fasting routine. Opt for:

- High-protein snacks: These can help keep you satiated longer, making it easier to stick to your fasting windows.
- Low-carb options: Choosing foods low in carbohydrates can help manage hunger and maintain energy levels by preventing blood sugar spikes and crashes.
- Fruits and vegetables: Rich in fibre and water, they're ideal for staying hydrated and full.

Adapting to New Rhythms

Flexibility is your ally when travelling across time zones or when your usual eating and fasting schedule doesn't align with travel plans. Consider:

- Adjust your fasting window: Shift your eating and fasting periods based on your travel schedule and activities. If you're crossing time zones, gradually adjust your fasting window a few days before your trip to align more closely with your destination's local time.
- Listen to your body: Travel can be taxing, and sometimes it's more beneficial to allow some leniency in your fasting schedule. If you find maintaining your usual fasting routine too challenging, it's okay to shorten your fasting windows or include more flexible eating periods during your trip.

In weaving through the challenges and opportunities that travel presents, what emerges is not just an adherence to a fasting regimen but an enriched experience of the world. Travelling while fasting encourages us to be more present, mindful of our choices, and adaptable to change. It's an invitation to explore not just new landscapes but also the depths of our discipline and flexibility.

As this exploration of intermittent fasting while travelling draws to a close, remember the key points that can make maintaining your fasting routine on the road not just feasible but also enjoyable. Preparation, smart food choices, and adaptability are your tools. They guide you in navigating the uncertainties of travel, ensuring that your commitment to fasting enhances rather than hampers your journey.

In the chapters that follow, we'll continue to unravel the layers of intermittent fasting, diving into the personal transformations it can foster. We'll see how the principles and practices we've explored become the foundation for lasting change, impacting not just our physical health but our entire approach to life and well-being.

Chapter 5: Clarity and Vitality: Unveiling the Mind's Potential Through Fasting

Intermittent Fasting: Transform Your Body and Mind

Imagine standing at the edge of a calm lake early in the morning, the surface so clear you can see to the depths below. This image mirrors the mental clarity and focus many experience through intermittent fasting. It's not just about clearing the fog; it's about peering into the depths of our cognitive abilities and tapping into a wellspring of mental sharpness that daily life often clouds.

In this chapter, we dive into how fasting acts like that quiet morning, settling the disturbances that obscure our mental clarity, and explore the mechanisms, practical applications, and real-life impacts of this fascinating benefit.

Enhancing Cognitive Function

The link between intermittent fasting and improved cognitive function is well-documented, with numerous studies pointing to sharper focus, better memory retention, and enhanced problem-solving abilities. It turns out that when we take a break from constantly feeding our bodies, we give our brains a unique kind of nourishment.

But why does this happen? During fasting, our bodies switch from using glucose to ketones as a primary energy source. Ketones, produced from the breakdown of fats, provide a more efficient and steady energy supply for the brain. This switch can lead to improved concentration and cognitive performance, essentially clearing the mental clutter to reveal a more focused mind.

Mechanisms Behind Mental Clarity

The science behind this mental boost is as fascinating as it is empowering. Two key players in this process are ketosis and reduced inflammation:

- Ketosis: Achieved during fasting, ketosis provides the brain with ketones, which are like high-octane fuel, supporting enhanced cognitive functions and neural growth.

Chapter 5: Clarity and Vitality: Unveiling the Mind's Potential Through Fasting

- Reduced Inflammation: Fasting reduces inflammation throughout the body, including the brain. Chronic inflammation is linked to cognitive decline, so this reduction can protect and improve brain health.

Understanding these processes can help us appreciate the profound impact fasting has beyond weight management, touching the very essence of how we think and process the world around us.

Practical Tips for Maximising Focus

With the why and how out of the way, let's get into the when and where—practical strategies for integrating fasting into your life to boost mental clarity:

1. Align demanding tasks with ketosis: Plan to tackle your most challenging projects during the peak times of ketosis in your fasting cycle, usually toward the end of the fasting period.
2. Stay hydrated: Dehydration can cloud your focus. Keep water close at hand, and don't hesitate to add a pinch of salt to replenish electrolytes, especially in longer fasting windows.
3. Mind your break-fast: When you do eat, choose foods that sustain cognitive energy. Think leafy greens, fatty fish, nuts, and seeds—all rich in brain-boosting nutrients like omega-3 fatty acids, antioxidants, and fibre.

Testimonials and Case Studies

While data and studies provide compelling evidence, hearing how intermittent fasting has changed lives offers a different kind of inspiration.

Consider the story of our good friend who is a programmer who found that intermittent fasting not only caused him to look and feel great but also brought a level of focus and creativity to his work previously unattainable. Coding sessions became more productive, solutions to complex problems more accessible, and the dreaded afternoon brain fog a thing of the past.

Or the account of a friend of my wife, a teacher who, after starting a 16/8 fasting schedule, noticed a significant improvement in memory recall and lesson planning. She reported that lessons became more engaging, student interactions more rewarding, and the overall sense of job satisfaction deepened.

These stories underline a common theme: intermittent fasting has the potential to enhance our mental faculties in profound ways, impacting our professional lives, personal projects, and everywhere in between.

Visual Element: Infographic on Brain-Boosting Foods for Break-Fast A colourful, engaging infographic that outlines the top foods to incorporate into your first meal after fasting to maximise cognitive benefits. This visual guide simplifies meal planning, ensuring your breakfast nourishes your brain as much as your body.

Interactive Element: Fasting Focus Tracker A simple, printable tracker designed to help you log your fasting schedule alongside daily focus and productivity levels. This tool enables you to visualise the correlation between your fasting periods and cognitive performance, guiding you to adjust for optimal mental clarity.

In wrapping up this exploration of fasting's impact on mental clarity and focus, it's clear that the practice offers more than just physical health benefits. It's a gateway to tapping into our cognitive potential, clearing the mental clutter, and enhancing our ability to think, learn, and create. Through understanding the mechanisms at play, implementing practical strategies for integrating fasting into our lives, and drawing inspiration from real-life transformations, we can begin to harness the full spectrum of benefits that intermittent fasting has to offer.

Chapter 5: Clarity and Vitality: Unveiling the Mind's Potential Through Fasting

5.2 The Energy Paradox: More Energy with Less Food

In a world where the norm often equates more food with more energy, intermittent fasting presents a curious contradiction. It suggests that by reducing our caloric intake during certain periods, we can boost our energy levels. This counterintuitive phenomenon—let's call it the energy paradox—stems from a fascinating interplay between our diet, our body's cellular mechanisms, and the ancient rhythms of feast and famine encoded in our DNA.

At the heart of this paradox lies the efficiency of our mitochondria, the powerhouses of our cells. When we fast, we give these tiny organelles a much-needed break from their constant battle with the byproducts of digestion and metabolism, allowing them to repair and become more efficient at converting nutrients into energy. This process is akin to tuning up an engine, resulting in a more efficient machine that runs smoother and lasts longer.

Balancing Macronutrients for Sustained Energy

The secret to unlocking sustained energy during your eating windows revolves around the strategic balance of macronutrients—carbohydrates, proteins, and fats. Each plays a unique role in fueling our bodies:

- Carbohydrates: Choose complex carbs, such as whole grains and vegetables, which offer a slow and steady release of glucose, keeping energy levels stable.
- Proteins: Including a good source of protein in your meals aids in muscle repair and growth, and it can also increase feelings of fullness, preventing energy dips.
- Fats: Healthy fats, found in foods like avocados, nuts, and olive oil, provide a dense energy source and support brain health, contributing to overall vitality.

Timing Meals for Energy Optimization

The timing of when we eat can be as crucial as what we eat, particularly when integrating fasting into our lifestyles. Here are some guidelines to help align your eating windows with your body's natural energy rhythms:

- Break the Fast Gently: Starting your day (or eating window) with a meal that includes a balance of macronutrients can jumpstart your metabolism and provide a steady energy source.
- Midday Meals: Aim for a lunch that includes a mix of complex carbs, protein, and healthy fats to maintain energy levels through the afternoon.
- Evening Eating: Consider a lighter meal to end your eating window, focusing on protein and vegetables to avoid sleep disturbances that could impact your energy the next day.

Personal Adjustments for Peak Energy

Finding your sweet spot when it comes to fasting lengths and eating windows requires a bit of experimentation. Here are some steps to fine-tune your approach:

1. Start Small: If you're new to fasting, begin with shorter fasting periods and gradually increase as your body adjusts.
2. Track Your Energy: Keep a log of your energy levels throughout the day, noting how different foods and meal timings affect your vitality.
3. Adjust as Needed: Use your energy log to make informed adjustments to your fasting schedule, meal composition, and timing.
4. Listen to Your Body: Pay close attention to how your body responds to changes in your fasting routine and be willing to adapt based on what you learn.

Chapter 5: Clarity and Vitality: Unveiling the Mind's Potential Through Fasting

This exploration of the energy paradox reveals that, paradoxically, less can indeed be more when it comes to food and energy. By understanding and utilising the underlying mechanisms of fasting, balancing our intake of macronutrients, and aligning our meals with our body's natural rhythms, we can unlock a level of energy and vitality that supports our active lives. Through mindful experimentation and a commitment to listening to our bodies, we pave the way for a more energised existence, fueled not by constant eating but by strategic nourishment and timing.

5.3 Autophagy: The Body's Natural Detox

Autophagy, a term derived from the Greek words for "self" (auto) and "eating" (phagy), is a process by which our cells clean the house. Think of it as the body's way of conducting a deep clean, getting rid of cellular debris like damaged proteins and organelles, and recycling parts that can be reused. This not only clears the way for new cellular growth and optimal function but also plays a crucial role in disease prevention and longevity.

At first glance, the idea that our cells essentially eat themselves to stay healthy might seem counterintuitive. However, this process is critical for maintaining cellular integrity and, by extension, our overall health. By removing damaged components, autophagy prevents bad proteins from accumulating and causing diseases. It's linked to reduced inflammation, a lower risk of neurodegenerative diseases, and even increased lifespan.

Fasting as a Trigger for Autophagy

While autophagy is a continuous process, certain conditions can accelerate it, with fasting being one of the most effective triggers. When we fast, the decrease in available nutrients forces our cells to find alternative sources of energy, leading to an increase in autophagy. Essentially, fasting prompts the body to "clean house," removing damaged cells and making room for new, healthy ones. This is not just theoretical; numerous studies have demonstrated that fasting increases autophagy in various tissues, contributing to improved health outcomes.

Different fasting regimes can initiate this process to varying degrees. Short-term fasts, like overnight or 24-hour fasts, begin the autophagic process, while longer fasts may enhance their depth and benefits. This doesn't mean one should jump straight into extended fasting periods. Even shorter, more frequent fasts can effectively boost autophagy, offering a practical and sustainable approach to harnessing this powerful cleansing mechanism.

Measuring Autophagy Effects

Measuring the effects of autophagy, especially in humans, poses a challenge. Most current research relies on markers found in laboratory tests, including changes in the levels of specific proteins associated with the autophagic process. For instance, an increase in the protein LC3-II and a decrease in p62/SQSTM1 are indicators of enhanced autophagy. While these markers provide valuable insights, the direct observation and measurement of autophagy in living organisms remain complex, requiring sophisticated techniques and technologies.

Despite these challenges, the evidence supporting the benefits of fasting-induced autophagy is compelling. Studies have shown that increased autophagy can lead to improved metabolic health, reduced risk of cancer, and enhanced longevity. As research methods evolve, we can expect to gain even deeper insights into how fasting influences autophagy and how we can optimise this process for health and longevity.

Balancing Autophagy and Nutrition

While the benefits of autophagy are clear, it's crucial to balance this process with adequate nutrition during eating periods. Supporting autophagy doesn't mean neglecting the body's need for essential nutrients. Here's how to strike that balance:

Chapter 5: Clarity and Vitality: Unveiling the Mind's Potential Through Fasting

- Prioritise nutrient-dense foods: When you do eat, focus on foods rich in vitamins, minerals, and antioxidants. Leafy greens, berries, nuts, and seeds can provide the raw materials your body needs for repair and growth.
- Protein is key: Adequate protein intake is essential for rebuilding and maintaining muscle mass, especially if you're engaging in strength training. Opt for high-quality sources like lean meats, fish, legumes, and dairy.
- Incorporate healthy fats: Fats, particularly omega-3 fatty acids found in fish and flaxseeds, support cell membrane health and can also promote brain function.
- Stay hydrated: Water is essential for all bodily functions, including autophagy. Ensure you're drinking enough throughout the day, especially during fasting periods.

By mindfully planning your eating windows to include a variety of nutrient-rich foods, you can support the body's natural detoxification process while ensuring you get the essential nutrients needed for optimal health. This approach allows you to reap the benefits of autophagy without compromising nutritional well-being, creating a foundation for a healthier, more vibrant life.

5.4 Fasting and Longevity: Adding Life to Your Years

The dance between fasting and longevity is a complex one, filled with nuances that researchers have been unravelling for years. At its core, the idea that abstaining from food for certain periods can not only enhance our present health but also add years to our lives is a concept that has captured the imagination of scientists and health enthusiasts alike. This section peers into the depths of how intermittent fasting could be the key to a longer, healthier life.

When we look at the connection between fasting and lifespan, the evidence is both compelling and intriguing. Studies have shown that intermittent fasting can lead to an extension of lifespan in various organisms, from simple yeasts to more complex mammals. This suggests that the benefits of fasting transcend the boundaries of species, hinting at universal biological mechanisms at play.

Mechanisms for Longevity

Several biological mechanisms are believed to contribute to the life-extending effects of fasting. Understanding these can help us appreciate the profound impact fasting can have on our health and longevity:

- Reduced Oxidative Stress: Fasting decreases the production of free radicals, and unstable atoms that can cause damage to cells, leading to ageing and disease. By reducing this oxidative stress, fasting helps preserve cellular health.
- Enhanced Metabolic Health: Fasting improves various metabolic markers, including insulin sensitivity, blood lipids, and blood sugar levels. These improvements reduce the risk of metabolic diseases, which are significant contributors to premature ageing.
- Increased Growth Hormone Secretion: Fasting triggers the secretion of growth hormone, which plays a role in fat metabolism and muscle growth. This hormone also has rejuvenating effects on tissues and organs, contributing to increased longevity.

The unfolding understanding of these mechanisms offers a glimpse into how fasting acts as a lever, pulling us toward a future of prolonged health and vitality.

Longevity Success Stories

Beyond the laboratory, real-world examples provide powerful testimony to the potential of fasting to enhance longevity. Cultures with dietary practices that incorporate fasting, such as those in Okinawa, Japan, and certain Mediterranean regions, often boast higher average

Chapter 5: Clarity and Vitality: Unveiling the Mind's Potential Through Fasting

lifespans. Here, fasting is not a trend but a way of life, woven into the fabric of their daily routines.

Individual stories further illuminate the impact of intermittent fasting on longevity. From individuals who have significantly improved their metabolic health and vigour to those who have reversed the markers of ageing, the anecdotes are as varied as they are inspiring. These narratives underscore the potential of fasting to not only add years to life but also life to years, enhancing the quality of life as we age.

Implementing Fasting for Long-Term Health

For those intrigued by the prospect of using fasting as a tool for longevity, several guidelines can help integrate this practice into life in a way that supports sustained health benefits:

- Start Slowly: Gradually introduce fasting into your routine, allowing your body to adjust. Begin with shorter fasting periods and slowly extend them as you become more comfortable.
- Prioritise Nutrition: During your eating periods, focus on nutrient-rich foods. A balanced diet that supports your fasting regimen is crucial for reaping the long-term benefits.
- Listen to Your Body: Pay attention to how your body responds to fasting. Adapt your fasting schedule as needed to align with your health goals and lifestyle.
- Stay Consistent: Consistency is key when it comes to fasting. Establish a routine that fits your life and stick with it, making adjustments as your needs and circumstances change.

By adopting intermittent fasting with these guidelines in mind, you can set a foundation for a lifestyle that supports not just a longer life, but a richer, healthier one as well.

The exploration of fasting's role in promoting longevity presents a compelling case for the integration of this ancient practice into modern life. Through a deeper understanding of the biological mechanisms at play, coupled with real-life success stories and practical implementation strategies, the potential of fasting to enhance our years becomes clear. This insight invites us to consider how intermittent fasting might not just change how we eat but also how we live, offering a pathway to a future marked by health, vitality, and longevity.

5.5 The Impact of Fasting on Inflammation

Inflammation is a natural response of the immune system, playing a crucial role in healing and protection against illness. However, when inflammation becomes chronic, it can act as a silent saboteur within the body, contributing to a host of chronic diseases. Interestingly, the practice of intermittent fasting offers a promising avenue for mitigating chronic inflammation, presenting a paradox where abstaining from food can lead to profound health benefits.

Reducing Chronic Inflammation Through Fasting

Intermittent fasting works on multiple fronts to dial down inflammation levels. It initiates a metabolic switch from glucose to ketones as an energy source, a transition that not only fuels the brain more efficiently but also reduces inflammatory markers. This switch, akin to shifting gears in a car to optimise performance, prompts the body to enter a state of cellular cleanup, removing debris and dysfunctional components that can drive inflammation.

Additionally, fasting periods help to recalibrate the immune system, reducing the production of pro-inflammatory cells and increasing the production of anti-inflammatory ones. This recalibration is akin to resetting a computer and clearing out glitches that cause the system to overreact.

Fasting Protocols for Anti-Inflammatory Effects

Not all fasting schedules are created equal, and some have shown more promise than others in reducing inflammation. Here are a few fasting protocols noted for their anti-inflammatory benefits:

Chapter 5: Clarity and Vitality: Unveiling the Mind's Potential Through Fasting

- Alternate Day Fasting: Alternating between days of normal eating and days of minimal calorie intake provides rhythmic stress on the body that strengthens cellular defences against inflammation.
- Time-Restricted Eating: Limiting the eating window each day, typically to 8-10 hours, aligns with the body's circadian rhythms, improving gut health and reducing systemic inflammation.
- Periodic Fasting: Engaging in extended fasts for 24-48 hours, though less frequently, can trigger significant anti-inflammatory responses by giving the body an extended break from digestion and allowing for deeper cellular repair.

Each of these methods introduces a pattern of eating that supports the body's natural anti-inflammatory processes, offering a tailored approach to reducing chronic inflammation based on individual lifestyles and health goals.

Dietary Considerations for Inflammation

What we choose to eat during our feeding windows can either amplify or diminish the anti-inflammatory benefits of fasting. Integrating anti-inflammatory foods into meals can bolster the body's defences against inflammation:

- Omega-3 Fatty Acids: Found in fish like salmon and plant sources such as flaxseeds, omega-3s are powerhouses in fighting inflammation.
- Antioxidant-Rich Foods: Berries, leafy greens, and nuts are loaded with antioxidants that neutralise free radicals, reducing oxidative stress and inflammation.
- Whole Grains: Rich in fibre, whole grains help maintain a healthy gut, which is crucial for controlling inflammation.
- Turmeric and Ginger: These spices contain compounds with potent anti-inflammatory effects, making them excellent additions to a wide array of dishes.

Incorporating these foods into your diet not only enhances the taste and variety of your meals but also leverages the synergistic effect of fasting and nutrition to combat inflammation.

Monitoring Inflammation Markers

Keeping an eye on inflammation levels can provide insights into how well your fasting regimen and dietary choices are working to reduce inflammation. Several markers and tests can help track these levels:

- C-reactive Protein (CRP): A blood test for CRP is one of the most commonly used markers to assess systemic inflammation.
- Erythrocyte Sedimentation Rate (ESR): This test measures how quickly red blood cells settle at the bottom of a test tube, with faster rates indicating more inflammation.
- Tumour Necrosis Factor-alpha (TNF-alpha) and Interleukin-6 (IL-6): Elevated levels of these cytokines in the blood are indicators of active inflammation.

Regular monitoring, ideally in coordination with a healthcare provider, can guide adjustments to your fasting and dietary strategies, ensuring they effectively address your inflammation-related health goals.

Navigating the complex relationship between fasting, diet, and inflammation requires a nuanced approach, blending periods of abstaining from food with thoughtful nutritional choices. By doing so, we tap into a powerful strategy for quelling chronic inflammation, setting the stage for a body less burdened by the risks of chronic diseases. This method of using intermittent fasting not only as a tool for weight management but also as a means to combat inflammation underscores the multifaceted benefits of this ancient practice, revealing its potential to significantly impact our health and well-being.

5.6 Fasting and Disease Prevention

In the realm of health and wellness, the potential of intermittent fasting to play a pivotal role in disease prevention has garnered significant

Chapter 5: Clarity and Vitality: Unveiling the Mind's Potential Through Fasting

attention. This method, characterised by periods of voluntary abstinence from food and drink, has been associated with a host of health benefits, notably in the prevention of chronic diseases such as heart disease, diabetes, and cancer. The evidence supporting these claims paints a picture of fasting not just as a tool for weight management, but as a key player in maintaining overall health and preventing disease.

Fasting for Cardiovascular Health

The heart, our most vital muscle, benefits greatly from the practice of intermittent fasting. Studies have shown that fasting can lead to improvements in several key factors related to heart health, including:

- Lowered Blood Pressure: Regular fasting has been linked to reductions in blood pressure, a major risk factor for heart disease.
- Improved Cholesterol Levels: Fasting can alter the lipid profile by decreasing the levels of LDL (bad) cholesterol and increasing HDL (good) cholesterol, helping to prevent plaque buildup in the arteries.
- Enhanced Arterial Health: Fasting encourages improved arterial function, reducing the risk of atherosclerosis, a condition characterised by hardened and narrowed arteries.

These changes contribute to a more robust cardiovascular system, mitigating the risk of heart disease and stroke, and underscoring the profound impact that fasting can have on heart health.

Fasting's Effect on Insulin Sensitivity and Diabetes Prevention

The rise of type 2 diabetes as a global health crisis has prompted a search for effective prevention strategies. Intermittent fasting emerges as a promising approach, primarily through its influence on insulin sensitivity. By periodically abstaining from food, our bodies are required to tap into stored glucose for energy, which in turn:

- Lowers Blood Sugar Levels: The utilisation of glucose during fasting periods helps to lower blood sugar levels, reducing the risk of developing diabetes.
- Improves Insulin Sensitivity: Regular fasting enhances the body's responsiveness to insulin, ensuring that glucose is efficiently removed from the blood and used by cells for energy.

This mechanism not only aids in the prevention of diabetes but also offers benefits for those already managing the condition, highlighting fasting's potential as a complementary approach to traditional diabetes care.

Potential for Fasting to Reduce Cancer Risk

The link between intermittent fasting and cancer prevention is a rapidly evolving area of research. Emerging studies suggest that fasting may exert a protective effect against cancer in a few key ways:

- Slowing Cell Growth: Fasting has been observed to slow down the rate of cell division, reducing the chances of cancerous mutations.
- Enhancing the Effectiveness of Cancer Treatments: Some research indicates that fasting can make cancer cells more susceptible to chemotherapy while protecting healthy cells, potentially improving treatment outcomes.

While the research is ongoing, the preliminary findings offer hope that intermittent fasting could play a role in cancer prevention and management, adding another layer to its multifaceted health benefits.

The exploration of intermittent fasting as a preventive measure against a spectrum of diseases reveals its potential beyond mere weight loss. By positively influencing heart health, enhancing insulin sensitivity, and possibly even reducing cancer risk, fasting presents a simple yet powerful lifestyle change that could significantly impact public health.

Chapter 5: Clarity and Vitality: Unveiling the Mind's Potential Through Fasting

As we conclude this section, it's clear that the implications of intermittent fasting extend far into the realms of disease prevention and health promotion. Its role in supporting cardiovascular health, preventing diabetes, and potentially reducing cancer risk underscores fasting's value as a versatile and accessible tool in our health arsenal.

Looking ahead, the journey into the world of intermittent fasting and its myriad benefits continues. The insights gained here pave the way for a deeper understanding of how this ancient practice can be harnessed in our modern lives, not just for disease prevention but for the enhancement of overall well-being. The next chapter builds on these foundations, exploring the practicalities of integrating fasting into daily life, ensuring that the benefits discussed here can be realised by anyone willing to embrace the fasting lifestyle.

Chapter 6: Adapt and Thrive: Intermittent Fasting Tailored for You

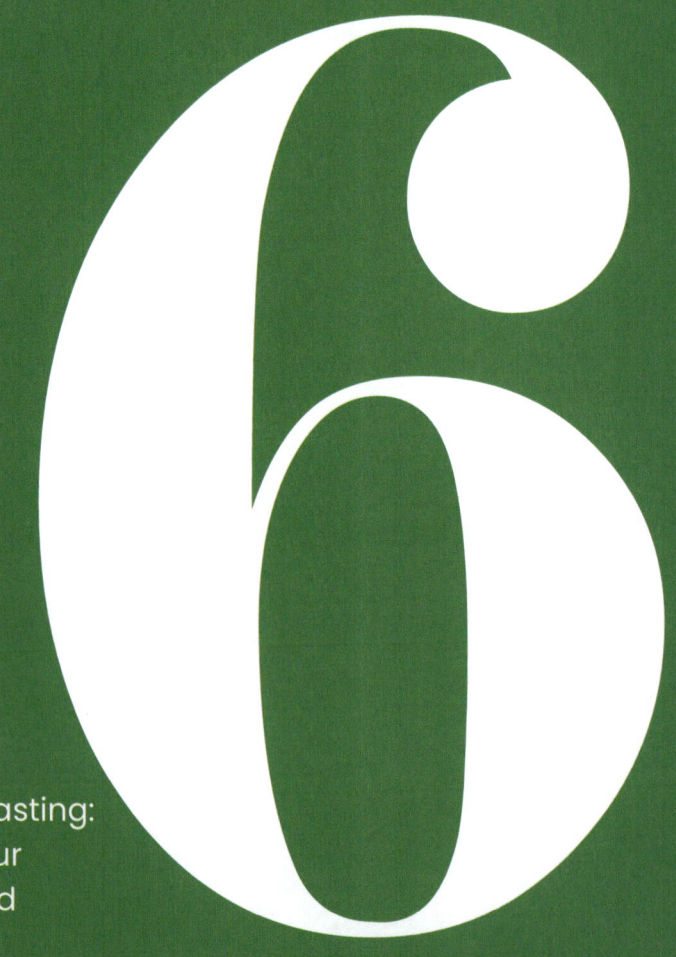

Chapter 6: Adapt and Thrive: Intermittent Fasting Tailored for You

The golden rays of dawn break the horizon, signalling not just the start of a new day but also the myriad possibilities that lie in personalising one's health regimen. Intermittent fasting, in its essence, is like clay - moldable, adaptable, and ready to be shaped to fit the contours of your unique life and body. This chapter delves into how intermittent fasting can be fine-tuned, focusing on the distinctive needs and considerations of women. It's about moving beyond the one-size-fits-all approach, recognizing the nuances that make each experience distinct, and addressing these with wisdom and care.

Intermittent Fasting for Women: Special Considerations

Understanding Hormonal Fluctuations

Women's bodies are rhythmic landscapes, shaped and reshaped by the ebb and flow of hormonal cycles. These cycles influence everything from energy levels to mood, and yes, how the body responds to fasting. The menstrual cycle, with its phases from follicular to luteal, impacts insulin sensitivity, metabolism, and hunger. Knowing this, it becomes clear that the fasting schedule that feels effortless one week might be a struggle the next. It's normal, and tweaking fasting times to match these hormonal rhythms can make all the difference.

Tailoring Fasting to Female Physiology

For women, the key to effective fasting lies in listening and adapting. For instance, during the luteal phase, when energy expenditure is higher and cravings are more intense, shortening fasting windows or even incorporating more nutrient-dense snacks can help maintain balance without derailing progress. On the other hand, the follicular phase might offer an opportunity to extend fasting periods comfortably. It's a dance of give and take, grounded in the understanding that flexibility doesn't mean inconsistency but rather a strategic response to the body's signals.

Fasting During Pregnancy and Breastfeeding

Pregnancy and breastfeeding are times of heightened nutritional demand, where the focus shifts to supporting not just the individual's health but also that of the baby. During these stages, intermittent fasting might need to take a back seat. However, principles of mindful eating and nutrient density - hallmarks of a well-structured fasting regimen - remain relevant. Consulting with healthcare professionals to craft a plan that nourishes both mother and child is paramount during these transformative periods.

Visual Element: Hormonal Phases and Fasting Guide

An infographic lays out the menstrual cycle's phases alongside tips for adjusting fasting schedules. It visually represents how insulin sensitivity, cravings, and energy levels fluctuate, providing a quick reference for women to align their fasting practices with their cycles.

Case Studies and Expert Opinions

Real-life experiences ground theory in reality, offering insights that are both relatable and inspiring. Conversations with healthcare professionals shed light on the nuances of intermittent fasting for women, highlighting the importance of a tailored approach. These narratives underscore a critical message: success in fasting, as in any health endeavour, comes from understanding and respecting the body's needs, crafting a regimen that supports these needs, and being open to adjustment.

Adjusting intermittent fasting to fit the unique aspects of women's health is not just about optimising results; it's about honouring the body's rhythms and requirements. It's a reminder that health practices are most effective when they are not imposed but grown from a deep understanding of oneself. This chapter invites women to embrace the flexibility that intermittent fasting offers, using it as a tool to enhance health while navigating the physiological changes that are inherent to their journey.

Chapter 6: Adapt and Thrive: Intermittent Fasting Tailored for You

6.2 Men and Fasting: What You Need to Know

Intermittent fasting has been shown to extend its benefits across the board, yet there are specific advantages that it brings to the table for men. To optimise health, fitness, and overall well-being, let's explore how this dietary pattern can be particularly beneficial for men, addressing common health concerns, and providing a roadmap to tailor fasting endeavours to meet personal health goals.

Benefits Specific to Men

In the realm of health and wellness, men often face unique challenges, including the risk of carrying excess abdominal fat and experiencing fluctuations in testosterone levels, both of which can have significant impacts on overall health. Intermittent fasting emerges as a powerful ally, offering benefits that are particularly salient for men:

- Enhanced Hormonal Balance: Fasting has been shown to positively influence hormonal health, including testosterone levels. Higher testosterone not only supports muscle growth and fat loss but also plays a crucial role in mood and libido.

- Muscle Maintenance and Growth: Unlike the misconception that fasting leads to muscle loss when coupled with resistance training, intermittent fasting can help men preserve and even build muscle, thanks to the increased human growth hormone levels.

- Efficient Fat Loss: Focusing on abdominal fat, intermittent fasting aids in targeting this stubborn area, promoting more efficient fat burning by improving metabolic rate and insulin sensitivity.

Addressing Men's Health Concerns

The spotlight on men's health brings to the forefront issues like heart disease, diabetes, and metabolic syndrome. Intermittent fasting steps in as a proactive measure, not just in managing but potentially preventing these conditions:

- Heart Health: Through the improvement of blood pressure, cholesterol levels, and arterial health, intermittent fasting contributes to a reduced risk of heart disease.
- Metabolic Enhancements: By aiding in weight management and enhancing insulin sensitivity, fasting supports metabolic health, offering a buffer against diabetes and metabolic syndrome.

Customising Fasting for Men's Health Goals

Tailoring an intermittent fasting schedule to fit individual health and fitness objectives ensures that the practice not only becomes sustainable but also maximally effective. Here are strategies to consider:

- Match Your Fasting Schedule to Your Lifestyle: Whether it's the 16/8 method or full 24-hour fasts, the key is finding a rhythm that aligns with your daily routine and physical activity levels.
- Incorporate Resistance Training: To maximise muscle maintenance and growth, schedule strength training sessions during your eating windows when you can fuel your muscles with protein-rich meals post-workout.
- Focus on Nutrient-Dense Foods: During eating periods, prioritise whole foods rich in proteins, healthy fats, and fibres to support testosterone levels and provide sustained energy.

Real-life Success Stories

Stories of transformation and triumph serve as a testament to the potential of intermittent fasting in men's lives. Consider my account. Middle-aged, facing the reality of creeping weight gain and declining energy, then I discovered intermittent fasting. Within months, not only did I shed the excess weight, but I also benefited from significant improvements in energy levels, mental clarity, and physical strength, a change that I attribute to a tailored fasting schedule and committed resistance training.

Chapter 6: Adapt and Thrive: Intermittent Fasting Tailored for You

Another narrative comes from a friend of mine who turned to intermittent fasting because he was inspired by the results I had. He is a professional who is at the top of his game but puts on lots of weight due to his busy schedule. He utilised fasting to manage stress and enhance focus at work. By aligning his fasting periods with his work schedule he found himself more alert, productive, and in control, highlighting the cognitive benefits that fasting brought into his life.

These stories underscore the versatility of intermittent fasting as a tool for men to not only confront health challenges but to elevate their quality of life. With each story, it becomes evident that when approached with intention and flexibility, intermittent fasting can significantly bolster men's health, fitness, and overall well-being.

6.3 Fasting During Menopause and Andropause

The midlife transition brings about significant changes, both physically and emotionally. For women, menopause marks the end of reproductive years, accompanied by a variety of symptoms ranging from hot flashes to mood swings. Men, although less discussed, experience andropause, characterised by a gradual decline in testosterone levels, affecting their energy, mood, and physical health. Intermittent fasting emerges not just as a dietary trend but as a tool that can be adapted to mitigate some of these changes, offering a way to navigate this phase with more ease and less discomfort.

Navigating Hormonal Changes with Fasting

The hormonal shifts during menopause and andropause can be challenging. Women may find weight management increasingly difficult due to a slowing metabolism and changes in body composition. Men might notice a decrease in muscle mass and an increase in abdominal fat. Intermittent fasting, with its metabolic and hormonal benefits, can be a powerful ally. By enhancing insulin sensitivity and promoting hormone balance, fasting helps manage weight and improve body composition. The key is to approach fasting with a flexible mindset, adjusting the duration and frequency to match one's changing needs and responses.

Adapting Fasting Methods for Midlife Transitions

Adapting fasting schedules to one's lifestyle and hormonal landscape can make intermittent fasting a sustainable practice during menopause and andropause. Here are some strategies:

- For women experiencing menopause, shorter fasting windows may mitigate feelings of fatigue and hunger, while still offering metabolic benefits. Incorporating more days of moderate fasting rather than a few days of more extended fasting can also be beneficial.
- Men going through andropause might find that maintaining muscle mass and managing weight becomes easier with time-restricted eating, particularly when eating periods align with times of physical activity.
- Both men and women could benefit from nutrient-dense foods during eating windows, focusing on proteins, healthy fats, and fibres to support hormonal health and satiety.

Personal Anecdotes and Guidance

Personal stories illuminate the path for those navigating fasting during menopause and andropause. Another friend of my wife shared how adjusting her fasting schedule to start later in the day helped manage her energy levels and reduce hot flashes. This lady's husband recounted how incorporating resistance training during his eating windows, coupled with a 16/8 fasting approach, aided in maintaining muscle mass and vitality.

These anecdotes highlight the importance of personalization and adaptation. What works for one person may not work for another, and the willingness to experiment and adjust is crucial.

Chapter 6: Adapt and Thrive: Intermittent Fasting Tailored for You

Expert Advice on Hormonal Health and Fasting

Healthcare professionals emphasise the importance of a holistic approach to fasting during these transitional periods. They recommend:

- Monitoring responses carefully and being willing to adjust fasting practices as needed. If sleep disturbances or mood swings increase, it might be worth shortening fasting periods or shifting the fasting window.

- Ensuring adequate nutrient intake during eating windows to support overall health, focusing on vitamins, minerals, and antioxidants that can bolster the body's response to hormonal changes.

- Staying hydrated and maintaining an active lifestyle complement the benefits of intermittent fasting and support overall well-being.

Incorporating intermittent fasting into one's lifestyle during menopause and andropause offers a way to actively manage some of the challenges these changes bring. It's not a magic bullet, but rather a tool that, when used thoughtfully and flexibly, can support health and well-being during a period of significant transition.

6.4 Intermittent Fasting with Medical Conditions

When navigating the waters of intermittent fasting while managing a chronic health condition, the primary beacon guiding this voyage should be collaboration with healthcare providers. This partnership is pivotal in tailoring a fasting program that not only respects the body's current state but also optimises health without exacerbating existing conditions. Here, we explore the nuances of fasting in the context of chronic health issues, offering insights into how adjustments might be necessary and highlighting instances where fasting might need to be approached with caution or possibly avoided.

Fasting with Chronic Conditions

Incorporating intermittent fasting into a routine complicated by chronic conditions such as diabetes, heart disease, or autoimmune disorders requires a careful, nuanced approach. It's not simply about the decision to fast but about how fasting integrates with overall health management strategies. For instance, individuals with diabetes need to monitor blood sugar levels closely, as fasting can significantly impact glucose control. Similarly, those with heart conditions should consider how changes in fluid and electrolyte balance during fasting periods might affect their health.

Modifying Fasting Plans for Health Challenges

Adjusting fasting schedules and dietary choices becomes essential when dealing with specific medical needs. Some adaptive strategies include:

- Shorter Fasting Windows: For those who might be at risk of adverse effects from longer fasting periods, starting with shorter fasting windows allows for the benefits of intermittent fasting without overwhelming the body.

- Nutrient-Dense Eating Windows: Ensuring that meals consumed during eating windows are rich in nutrients supports overall health and can help manage chronic conditions more effectively. It involves focusing on whole foods, lean proteins, healthy fats, and plenty of fruits and vegetables.

- Regular Monitoring: Keeping a close watch on how the body responds to fasting, with particular attention to any health markers relevant to chronic conditions, enables timely adjustments to the fasting plan.

Case Studies of Fasting with Medical Conditions

The stories of individuals who have navigated intermittent fasting alongside managing chronic health conditions shed light on

Chapter 6: Adapt and Thrive: Intermittent Fasting Tailored for You

the practicality and potential of fasting in these contexts. One case involves a person with type 2 diabetes who, under medical supervision, adopted an intermittent fasting schedule. This individual reported improved blood sugar control and reduced reliance on medication, attributing success to careful planning, regular monitoring, and close communication with their healthcare provider.

Another case highlights the experience of someone with rheumatoid arthritis, a chronic autoimmune condition characterised by inflammation and pain. Through intermittent fasting, they noticed a decrease in inflammation markers and an improvement in joint mobility. Key to their success was a focus on anti-inflammatory foods during eating windows and gradual adjustments to fasting durations, based on how their body responded.

When to Avoid Fasting

While intermittent fasting offers numerous health benefits, there are circumstances and conditions where fasting might not be advisable. Recognizing these scenarios is crucial for safety and overall well-being:

- Severe Metabolic Disorders: Individuals with severe metabolic diseases, such as advanced liver or kidney diseases, should exercise caution, as fasting could potentially exacerbate these conditions.

- Eating Disorders: For those with a history of eating disorders, fasting can trigger unhealthy patterns and behaviours. In these cases, other health strategies might be more appropriate.

- Pregnancy and Breastfeeding: As previously mentioned, the nutritional demands during pregnancy and breastfeeding are heightened. Fasting could compromise nutrient intake, affecting both maternal and child health.

The journey of integrating intermittent fasting into a lifestyle complicated by chronic health conditions underscores the importance of personalised health strategies. It highlights that with thoughtful adjustments, regular monitoring, and, most importantly, partnership with healthcare professionals, intermittent fasting can be a valuable component of managing and potentially improving chronic health issues.

6.5 When to Pause: Listening to Your Body's Signals

In the unfolding narrative of our lives, where intermittent fasting becomes a protagonist in our quest for health, there stand moments that whisper for a pause. The art of fasting isn't merely about adherence to schedules but an ongoing conversation with our bodies, a dialogue that respects the cues and signs necessitating a gentle halt or a thoughtful adjustment. This chapter shines a light on recognizing these moments, understanding the intrinsic value of flexibility, navigating the interlude of a pause, and resuming with renewed insight.

Recognizing Signs to Take a Break

Our bodies communicate in subtle ways, signalling when it's time to ease off or momentarily step away from fasting. These signals can manifest both physically and mentally, deserving our attention and action. Physical signs might include unusual fatigue, persistent hunger that goes beyond the normal adjustment period, or disruptions in sleep patterns that leave us tossing and turning into the night. Mentally, a constant preoccupation with food, feelings of irritability, or a noticeable dip in concentration can also indicate the need for a pause. Acknowledging these signs isn't a step back but a necessary act of self-care, ensuring our fasting practices align with our body's needs.

Importance of Flexibility in Fasting

The landscape of our lives is ever-changing, with each day presenting its own set of challenges and demands. Flexibility in our fasting regimen isn't just beneficial; it's essential for weaving this practice into the fabric of our daily existence without fraying the edges. This adaptability ensures that fasting enhances our lives without becoming a source of additional stress. It allows us to adjust our fasting windows around life events, fluctuating work schedules, or shifts in our

Chapter 6: Adapt and Thrive: Intermittent Fasting Tailored for You

physical and emotional well-being, making fasting a sustainable and enriching part of our routine.

Strategies for Pausing and Resuming Fasting

Navigating the waters of a pause in fasting involves more than merely breaking the fast; it's about maintaining a conscious connection with our nutritional needs and intentions. Here are strategies to transition into and out of a fasting pause:

- Introduce Light Meals: If you decide to pause, start with light meals that are easy on digestion. Soups, salads, and smoothies can provide nourishment without overwhelming your system.
- Stay Hydrated: Continuing to drink plenty of water during a break helps maintain hydration levels and supports overall health.
- Mindful Eating: Use the pause to engage in mindful eating practices, savouring each bite and paying attention to hunger and fullness cues, which can be enlightening when you resume fasting.
- Gradual Resumption: When you feel ready to reintroduce fasting, start with shorter windows and gradually extend them as your body readjusts. This gradual approach reduces the likelihood of discomfort and makes the transition smoother.

Listening and responding to your body during these times fortify the relationship you have with yourself, fostering a practice that truly aligns with your well-being.

Listening to Your Body's Feedback

At its heart, intermittent fasting is a personal journey of discovery, one that requires tuning in to the body's feedback and responding with kindness and adjustment. This attentiveness involves more than observing physical reactions; it's about aligning our fasting practice with our internal rhythms and life demands. Keeping a journal can be an insightful tool for tracking how different fasting schedules impact energy levels, sleep quality, mood, and overall health. This record becomes a map, guiding adjustments and illuminating the path to a fasting rhythm that resonates with our individual needs and goals.

In this continuous cycle of listening, pausing, and adjusting, we find not just the key to a sustainable fasting practice but also to a deeper understanding of ourselves. It's a testament to the idea that sometimes, to move forward with greater strength and clarity, we must allow ourselves the grace to pause, reflect, and proceed with renewed purpose.

6.6 Fasting and Medications: A Guide

Navigating the waters of intermittent fasting while on medication requires thoughtful consideration of how the two might interact. It's not uncommon for fasting to influence how the body metabolises various drugs, and vice versa, medications can impact the effectiveness and experience of fasting. This delicate balance calls for a proactive approach, prioritising open discussions with healthcare professionals to tailor a fasting regimen that complements medical treatments.

How Fasting Affects Medication Responses

The body's absorption and processing of medication can shift during fasting periods. For some, fasting may slow down the rate at which medications are metabolised, potentially altering their effectiveness. For others, particularly with medications that rely on food for proper absorption, fasting could diminish their efficacy. It's also worth noting that fasting can influence hydration levels, further affecting medication absorption and processing.

The Imperative of Healthcare Consultation

Before adjusting your eating patterns, initiating a conversation with your healthcare provider is critical. This dialogue should encompass the specifics of your medication regimen, any known interactions with changes in diet or fasting, and the potential need for dosage adjustments. It's also an opportunity to discuss how fasting might align with your overall health strategy, ensuring that your approach supports your wellness goals without compromising medical treatment.

Chapter 6: Adapt and Thrive: Intermittent Fasting Tailored for You

Timing Fasting Schedules Around Medications

When medications need to be taken with food, crafting your fasting schedule to accommodate this requirement becomes an essential strategy. Some find success by aligning their eating window with the timing of their medication, ensuring they can take their doses as prescribed without breaking their fast unexpectedly. This might mean adjusting the start or end times of your fasting window or possibly adopting a fasting method that offers greater flexibility, like the 12-hour fast, which can more easily accommodate medication schedules.

Monitoring Your Health While Fasting on Medication

Keeping a close eye on how your body responds to fasting while on medication is crucial. This vigilance helps in identifying any changes in how you feel or how effectively your medications seem to be working. Regular check-ins with your healthcare provider, coupled with self-monitoring of any symptoms or changes, provide a feedback loop that can guide necessary adjustments to your fasting or medication regimen. Tools such as blood pressure monitors, glucose metres, or symptom diaries can be invaluable in this process, offering concrete data to share with your healthcare team.

In stepping into the realm of intermittent fasting while managing medication, the journey becomes one of careful navigation, informed by open communication with healthcare professionals and attentive self-monitoring. This path is not about choosing between fasting and effective medical treatment but finding how the two can coexist, each supporting the other in fostering your health and well-being.

As we wrap up this exploration, the guiding principles that emerge underscore the importance of informed, personalised approaches to integrating fasting into our lives, especially when medications are part of our health landscape. The dialogue with healthcare providers, thoughtful scheduling, and vigilant monitoring form the pillars of a fasting practice that respects our body's needs and the role of medications in maintaining our health. These considerations pave the way for a fasting experience that enriches our journey towards wellness, embodying a holistic view that sees beyond the confines of diet to embrace the full spectrum of healthful living.

Chapter 7: **Nourishing Your Fasting Lifestyle**

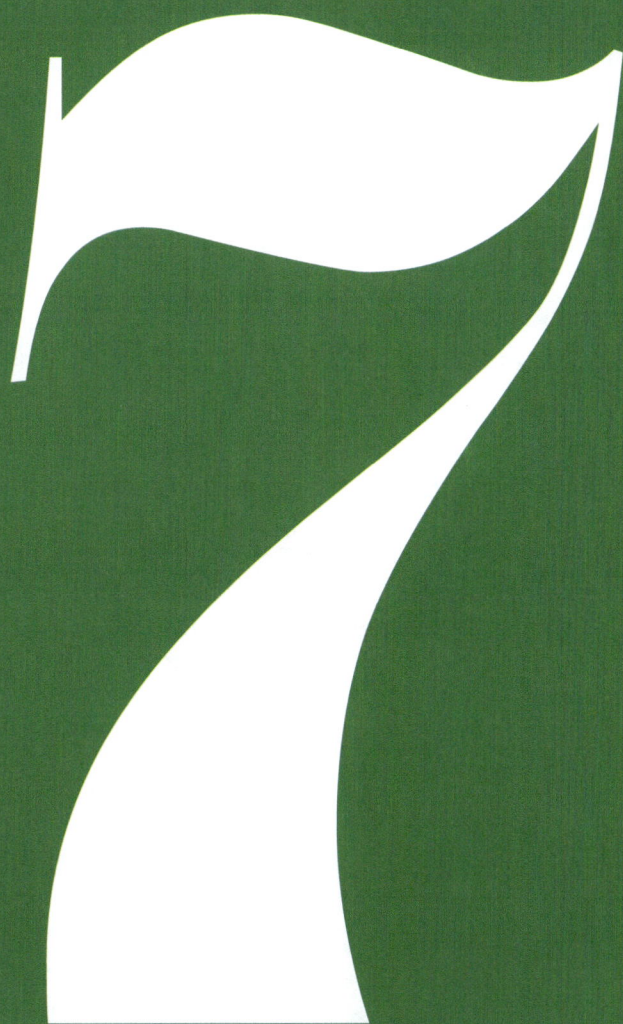

Intermittent Fasting: Transform Your Body and Mind

Imagine your body as a finely tuned instrument. The food you consume is the melody you play, and intermittent fasting is the rhythm that brings harmony to the performance. Crafting your intermittent fasting meal plan isn't just about deciding what or when to eat; it's about creating a symphony that resonates with your body's needs, activity levels, and personal goals. This chapter turns the spotlight on how to compose your unique dietary score, ensuring every note contributes to your well-being.

Balancing Macronutrients

A well-composed meal plan strikes a perfect chord between proteins, fats, and carbohydrates. Each macronutrient plays a vital role:

- Proteins are the building blocks, repairing tissues and muscles, especially crucial after workouts.
- Fats are like a steady rhythm, providing long-lasting energy and supporting cell function.
- Carbohydrates act as quick, bright notes, offering immediate energy and supporting brain function.

Imagine packing a lunch box for a day out. You'd include a mix of nuts for healthy fats, a chicken wrap for protein, and a serving of quinoa salad rich in complex carbs. This combination ensures you have sustained energy and nutrients for recovery, no matter your plans.

Considering Nutrient Density

Choosing nutrient-dense foods is like opting for high-quality instruments; they ensure better performance and longevity. Nutrient-dense foods pack a significant amount of vitamins, minerals, and other beneficial compounds into each calorie, offering more nourishment per bite. This means vibrant salads packed with leafy greens, colourful berries bursting with antioxidants, and fatty fish rich in omega-3s. When planning meals, think of incorporating a rainbow of colours from fruits and vegetables, ensuring you're not just eating, but nourishing your body.

Chapter 7: Nourishing Your Fasting Lifestyle

Aligning Meals with Activity Levels

Timing your meals to sync with your activity levels maximises energy use and recovery. On days filled with meetings or desk-bound tasks, a lighter menu might suffice, focusing on salads, soups, and lean proteins. Conversely, before a long run or a heavy lifting session, a meal richer in complex carbohydrates will fuel your endurance and performance. Post-workout, a protein-centric dish aids in muscle repair. Imagine scheduling a big meal for lunch before an afternoon of hiking. It fuels your adventure, ensuring you have the energy to enjoy every moment.

Personalising Your Meal Plan

Tailoring your meal plan acknowledges that you are unique. Your age, health conditions, taste preferences, and goals all play into what an ideal meal plan looks like for you. For someone managing diabetes, focusing on low-glycemic foods that stabilise blood sugar is crucial. If you're aiming to build muscle, upping protein and caloric intake during eating windows becomes a priority. And let's not forget about taste—enjoying what you eat is just as important. Love spicy food? Adding chilli peppers to dishes can boost metabolism. Adore sweets? Incorporating natural sweeteners and fruit can satisfy those cravings without derailing your progress.

Visual Element: The Balanced Plate Infographic

A vibrant infographic titled "The Balanced Plate" shows how to portion your plate according to macronutrients for different goals: weight loss, muscle gain, and maintenance. It visualises the ideal balance of proteins, fats, and carbs, with examples of foods for each category, making meal planning a visual and intuitive process.

Crafting your intermittent fasting meal plan is a dynamic process, one that evolves as you tune into your body's responses and discover what works best for you. It's about nourishment, enjoyment, and alignment with your lifestyle and goals, creating a dietary rhythm that not only supports your fasting journey but enhances your overall quality of life.

7.2 Quick and Nutritious Recipes for Your Eating Window

Breaking your fast is like greeting the morning sun after a peaceful night's slumber. You want that first ray of light to be gentle yet invigorating, preparing you for the day ahead. The same principle applies to the meals that reintroduce your body to nourishment. Let's explore recipes designed to replenish, energise, and satisfy, making each eating window an opportunity to nourish your body and delight your taste buds.

Breakfast Meals

The first meal of your day sets the tone for how you will feel and perform. Aim for options that are kind to your digestive system while providing essential nutrients to break your fast gently:

- Avocado and Egg Toast on Sprouted Grain Bread
- Mash half an avocado and spread it on toasted sprouted grain bread.
- Top with a poached egg, a sprinkle of red pepper flakes, and a dash of sea salt.
- The healthy fats in the avocado, combined with the high-quality protein from the egg, offer a balanced start, while the sprouted grain bread introduces complex carbohydrates slowly.
- Smoothie with Spinach, Blueberries, and Plant Protein
- Blend a handful of spinach, half a cup of blueberries, one scoop of your preferred plant protein powder, a tablespoon of flaxseeds, and almond milk.
- This smoothie is a powerhouse of antioxidants, omega-3 fatty acids, and protein. It's an excellent liquid meal that's easy on your stomach but packed with nutrients.

Chapter 7: Nourishing Your Fasting Lifestyle

High-energy Meals

For days when your calendar is packed with back-to-back activities or you're gearing up for a workout, high-energy meals that fuel your body and mind are non-negotiable:

- Quinoa Salad with Roasted Chickpeas and Vegetables
- Combine cooked quinoa with roasted chickpeas, diced peppers, cucumbers, cherry tomatoes, and a lemon-tahini dressing.
- Quinoa and chickpeas provide a solid protein and carbohydrate base, ensuring sustained energy, while the vegetables keep the meal light and hydrating.
- Turkey and Hummus Wrap
- Spread hummus on a whole wheat wrap, and add slices of roast turkey, cucumbers, shredded carrots, and lettuce. Roll tightly.
- The lean protein from the turkey, complex carbs from the wrap, and fibre from the vegetables create a balanced meal that's satisfying yet energising.

Satisfying Dinners

As the day winds down, a fulfilling dinner that comforts without overloading your digestive system ensures a restful night. These meals strike a perfect balance between satisfying your hunger and supporting your fasting goals:

- Grilled Salmon with Sweet Potato and Asparagus
- Grill a salmon fillet and serve with a baked sweet potato and grilled asparagus.
- Salmon provides omega-3 fatty acids, crucial for brain health, while sweet potato and asparagus offer a comforting yet light side that aids in overnight fasting.
- Stuffed Bell Peppers

- Stuff halved bell peppers with a mixture of ground turkey, cooked quinoa, diced tomatoes, and spices. Bake until the peppers are tender.
- This dish is visually appealing and nutritionally balanced, offering a variety of textures and flavours to keep dinner exciting.

Healthy Treats

Satisfying a sweet tooth without derailing your fasting progress is possible with treats that are as nutritious as they are delicious:

- Almond Butter and Banana Rice Cakes
- Spread almond butter on brown rice cakes and top with banana slices and a sprinkle of cinnamon.
- This snack offers a quick, satisfying fix to sweet cravings with the added benefit of healthy fats and potassium.
- Dark Chocolate and Nut Clusters
- Melt dark chocolate and mix in a handful of almonds, walnuts, and a sprinkle of sea salt. Drop spoonfuls onto a parchment paper and cool until set.
- Dark chocolate is rich in antioxidants, while nuts provide a crunch and a dose of healthy fats, making these clusters a guilt-free treat.

Each recipe in this section is crafted to align with the principles of intermittent fasting, ensuring that your meals support your health goals while satisfying your culinary cravings. From the gentle welcome of break-fast meals to the comforting embrace of dinner and the delightful indulgence of healthy treats, these recipes are designed to nourish, energise, and delight, making every eating window an opportunity to celebrate food in its most nutritious and delicious forms.

7.3 Preparing Meals in Advance: Batch Cooking and Storage Tips

In the rhythm of life where intermittent fasting plays its tune, preparing meals in advance harmonises your dietary needs with your bustling schedule. This section introduces you to the art of batch cooking, effective food storage, and the integration of meal prep into your fasting regimen, complemented by a list of kitchen gadgets designed to make healthy cooking a breeze.

Batch Cooking Strategies

Crafting a week's worth of meals in one cooking session might sound like a symphony requiring a full orchestra, but with a bit of orchestration, you'll find the melody is surprisingly simple. Here's how to conduct your batch cooking:

- Plan Your Menu: Start by selecting recipes that share ingredients to streamline your shopping list and minimise waste. Think of a savoury chicken that can serve as the protein in salads, wraps, or paired with roasted vegetables.
- Cook in Stages: Begin with foods requiring longer cooking times, such as roasts or stews. While these simmer or bake, you can prepare quicker dishes or chop vegetables for salads and snacks.
- Make It Fun: Turn on your favourite music or podcast to keep the atmosphere light and enjoyable as you cook.

Batch cooking isn't just about efficiency; it's a ritual that sets the stage for a week of nourishing, fasting-friendly meals, ensuring you always have something healthy and satisfying at hand.

Proper Food Storage

Once the cooking crescendo fades, storing your culinary creations correctly ensures they retain their freshness and nutritional value until you're ready to enjoy them. Here are some guidelines:

- Cool Before Storing: Allow cooked foods to cool to room temperature before refrigerating or freezing to prevent moisture buildup, which can lead to spoilage.

- Use Airtight Containers: Invest in quality airtight containers in various sizes. Glass containers are ideal for visibility and avoiding unwanted chemicals leaching into your food.
- Label and Date: Mark each container with the contents and the date it was cooked. This not only helps you keep track of freshness but also makes meal selection easier during your eating window.

Proper storage is the encore to your batch cooking performance, ensuring that each meal is as delightful as when it was first prepared.

Meal Prep for Busy Schedules

Incorporating meal prep into your fasting schedule can seem daunting amidst life's cacophony. Yet, with a bit of planning, it becomes a seamless part of your routine:

- Align Prep with Your Fasting Window: Choose a day and time for meal prep that falls within your eating window, allowing you to taste-test dishes as needed.
- Create a Meal Calendar: Sketch out your meals for the week, considering your fasting/eating schedule, workout days, and any social plans that might affect your meal choices.
- Prep Components Instead of Whole Meals: Consider preparing versatile components like grilled proteins, roasted vegetables, and whole grains. These can be mixed and matched to create varied meals on the fly.

Meal prep isn't just about having food ready; it's about creating a buffer against the unexpected, ensuring that even on the busiest days, you can maintain your fasting and eating rhythm without missing a beat.

Time-Saving Kitchen Tools

To make the process of meal prep both efficient and enjoyable, certain tools can prove invaluable. Here's a list of kitchen gadgets that can expedite your meal preparation process:

- High-Quality Knives: A set of sharp, durable knives makes chopping and slicing not only faster but safer.
- Slow Cooker or Instant Pot: These appliances are perfect for making large batches of stews, soups, and roasts with minimal hands-on time.
- Food Processor: Ideal for quickly chopping vegetables, grinding nuts and seeds, or making sauces and dressings.
- Silicone Baking Mats and Parchment Paper: These non-stick surfaces make cleanup a breeze, especially after roasting vegetables or baking.
- Measuring Cups and Spoons: Essential for ensuring consistency in your recipes, especially when you're dividing meals into portions.

Equipping your kitchen with these tools turns meal prep from a daunting chore into a swift and satisfying prelude to your week, allowing you more time to savour the moments that matter.

In weaving these strategies into the fabric of your intermittent fasting lifestyle, you create a tapestry of preparedness and healthful eating. Batch cooking, coupled with effective storage and strategic meal prep, ensures that your nourishment is always in harmony with your dietary rhythms, making every meal a note in the melody of your well-being.

7.4 Smart Snacking: What to Eat and When

In the realms of both music and meals, timing and composition are everything. This holds not just for the grand symphonies of our main meals but also for the brief interludes of snacks that punctuate our days. Within your eating window, these snacks play a crucial role, ensuring that energy remains high and cravings stay low, all while keeping true to the principles of intermittent fasting.

Choosing Fasting-Friendly Snacks

The art of snacking while adhering to an intermittent fasting schedule demands a keen eye for nutrient density and a commitment to satiety. The ideal snack is more than just a stopgap; it's a carefully chosen mini-meal that sustains you without disrupting your fasting benefits. Look for options that combine fibres, proteins, and healthy fats:

- Fibre-rich vegetables, such as carrots or bell peppers, dipped in guacamole, offer a crunchy way to fill up and fuel up.
- Greek yoghurt with a sprinkle of chia seeds serves as a protein-packed base, enhanced with omega-3 fatty acids for extended energy release.

These choices keep you satiated, making it easier to maintain your fasting schedule without feeling deprived or overly hungry before your next meal.

Timing Snacks for Energy

The strategic placement of snacks within your eating window can elevate your energy levels and ensure you're firing on all cylinders throughout the day. The goal is to distribute your intake so that you experience consistent energy, avoiding the peaks and troughs that can come from less thoughtful eating. Consider:

- Have a mid-morning snack, such as a handful of nuts and seeds, if your eating window begins in the morning. This provides a slow release of energy and keeps hunger at bay.
- If your window stretches into the evening, a late-afternoon snack of Greek yoghurt can bridge the gap to dinner without weighing you down.

This approach to timing helps maintain a steady stream of energy, supporting both physical activity and mental acuity without leading to spikes in hunger.

Chapter 7: Nourishing Your Fasting Lifestyle

Snacking vs. Meal Frequency

In the tapestry of your daily eating plan, it's crucial to distinguish between effective snacking and inadvertently increasing meal frequency. The latter can inadvertently turn into a series of mini-meals that edge you away from the fasting-focused benefits you're aiming for. To navigate this:

- Limit snacks to one or two per eating window, ensuring they're planned and purposeful rather than impulsive.
- Focus on hydration—sometimes thirst masquerades as hunger. A glass of water before reaching for a snack can clarify whether you're genuinely hungry.
- Space snacks and meals thoughtfully, allowing time for digestion and absorption, and preventing a continuous cycle of eating that can negate the effects of fasting.

Adopting this mindful approach ensures that snacks serve their purpose as energising interludes rather than becoming unintentional extensions of your meals.

Healthy Snack Recipes

Creating snacks that satisfy without derailing your fasting efforts is both an art and a science. Here are a couple of recipes that blend flavour, nutrition, and simplicity, proving that snacking can be both delicious and fasting-friendly:

- Apple Slices with Almond Butter
- Thinly slice an apple and spread a thin layer of almond butter on each slice.
- The crispness of the apple paired with the creamy richness of almond butter provides a satisfying snack that's rich in fibre and healthy fats.
- Cucumber and Hummus Boats

- Slice a cucumber into long halves and scoop out the seeds to create a groove.
- Fill each groove with hummus and sprinkle with paprika for a refreshing snack that combines hydration with protein and fibre.

These recipes embody the perfect snacking philosophy for intermittent fasters: nutrient-dense, satisfying, and simple. They're designed to slot seamlessly into your eating window, providing energy and fulfilment without complexity or excess.

In navigating the world of snacking within the intermittent fasting framework, the emphasis on nutrient density, strategic timing, and mindfulness ensures that these smaller culinary moments enrich your fasting experience. They become not just moments of sustenance but opportunities to enhance your health, energy, and enjoyment of the fasting lifestyle, all while keeping you on track toward your goals.

7.5 Hydration and Intermittent Fasting: Best Practices

Maintaining optimal hydration is a cornerstone of health, more so when intermittent fasting. While the act of fasting inherently focuses on when and what we eat, how we drink—what, when, and how much—merits equal attention. This section sheds light on hydration's pivotal role in fasting and offers insights for integrating it seamlessly into your fasting regimen.

The Pivotal Role of Hydration in Fasting

When you fast, your body undergoes several physiological changes, one of which is a shift in how fluids and electrolytes are managed. Given that a significant portion of daily fluid intake typically comes from food, fasting can inadvertently lead to reduced hydration if not consciously managed. This is especially true during prolonged fasts or in warmer climates, where the body's demand for water increases. Staying hydrated ensures that your metabolism functions smoothly, aids in the removal of toxins, and helps curb hunger pangs that might be mistaken for thirst.

Hydration extends beyond simply drinking water. It's about maintaining a balance of fluids and electrolytes that support your body's needs. When fasting, the significance of this balance cannot be overstated, as it impacts everything from cognitive function to physical performance and overall well-being.

Exploring Hydration Sources Beyond Water

While water is the most straightforward way to stay hydrated, fasting offers an opportunity to explore other hydrating beverages that can add variety and additional benefits:

- Herbal Teas: Herbal teas, served hot or iced, can be a comforting way to increase your fluid intake. Options like chamomile can soothe the digestive system, while peppermint tea may alleviate hunger pangs.

- Electrolyte-Infused Drinks: Especially after workouts or in hot weather, drinks enhanced with electrolytes can help replenish what's lost through sweat. Opt for versions without added sugars or artificial sweeteners.

- Bone Broth: For those practising a fasting regimen that allows for some caloric intake during fasting windows, sipping on bone broth can provide hydration along with essential minerals.

- Infused Water: Adding slices of fruits or cucumbers to water not only enhances flavour but can also encourage you to drink more throughout the day.

These alternatives to plain water not only keep you hydrated but also support your fasting experience, making it more enjoyable and sustainable.

Recognizing and Managing Hydration Status

Staying vigilant about your hydration status is key to avoiding dehydration. Familiarise yourself with the signs that might indicate you need to up your fluid intake:

- Feeling Thirsty: Thirst is the body's direct signal that it needs more fluids. Don't ignore it.
- Changes in Urine: Dark urine or a decrease in frequency can be indicators of dehydration.
- Dry Mouth or Bad Breath: A dry mouth or an unusual taste can signal a need for more water.
- Fatigue or Dizziness: These can both be signs that your body is lacking fluids.
- By paying close attention to these signals, you can proactively manage your hydration, ensuring that your fasting journey is both effective and healthful.

Seamlessly Integrating Hydration into Your Fasting Plan

Strategically incorporating fluids into your fasting and eating windows can help maintain optimal hydration levels without feeling overwhelmed. Here are practical tips for doing just that:

- Start and End Your Day with Water: Begin your day with a tall glass of water to replenish fluids lost overnight. Similarly, ending your eating window with water can help sustain hydration levels during your fast.
- Carry a Water Bottle: Keeping water on hand at all times makes it easier to sip throughout the day, rather than trying to catch up all at once.
- Set Hydration Reminders: In the hustle and bustle of daily life, drinking water can slip our minds. Setting reminders on your phone or computer can help maintain a steady intake.
- Hydrate Based on Activity Level: Adjust your fluid intake on days you're more active or when the weather is warmer to compensate for increased fluid loss.

Chapter 7: Nourishing Your Fasting Lifestyle

- Listen to Your Body: Just as with eating, listen to your body's cues for hydration. If you're feeling thirsty, drink up, regardless of where you are in your fasting or eating window.

Fluids play a critical role in not just surviving but thriving during intermittent fasting. By varying your sources of hydration, staying alert to your body's hydration signals, and thoughtfully integrating fluids into your fasting regimen, you can enhance your fasting experience, bolster your health, and ensure that every day of fasting brings you closer to your wellness goals.

7.6 Supplements: Enhancing Your Fasting Experience

In the realm of intermittent fasting, while the primary focus often lands squarely on what and when we eat, the role of supplements to bolster our nutritional intake can't be overlooked. Navigating the world of vitamins and minerals adds another layer to optimising your fasting regimen, ensuring your body receives the full spectrum of nutrients it needs to function at its best.

Identifying Supplemental Needs

The first step in integrating supplements into your fasting lifestyle involves assessing whether your current diet, in conjunction with your fasting schedule, meets your nutritional needs. This assessment should take into account not only the variety and quantity of foods you consume but also specific health goals or concerns. For instance, if your eating window restricts the inclusion of certain food groups, or if you have underlying health conditions that affect nutrient absorption, supplements can help fill those gaps.

Consider keeping a food diary for a few weeks, tracking what you eat and any physical or mental changes you notice. This record can be instrumental in identifying patterns or deficiencies that supplements could address. Additionally, blood tests can offer concrete insights into any specific nutrients your body may be lacking.

Best Supplements for Fasters

Depending on your dietary intake and health objectives, certain supplements stand out for their universal benefits, especially for individuals practising intermittent fasting:

- Multivitamins: A quality multivitamin acts as a nutritional safety net, covering a broad spectrum of vitamins and minerals that might be missing from your diet.
- Omega-3 Fatty Acids: Essential for heart and brain health, omega-3 supplements, such as fish oil or algae oil for vegetarians, support anti-inflammatory processes and cognitive function.
- Electrolytes: Magnesium, potassium, and sodium are crucial for hydration, nerve function, and muscle contraction. Supplementing with electrolytes can be particularly beneficial during longer fasting periods to maintain electrolyte balance.
- Vitamin D: Given its importance for bone health, immune function, and mood regulation, and considering the challenge of obtaining sufficient vitamin D from food alone, a vitamin D supplement is often recommended, especially for those in less sunny climates.

Incorporating these supplements can help ensure your body doesn't just survive but thrives during fasting, supporting overall health and well-being.

Timing Supplement Intake

Maximising the benefits of supplements while fasting involves strategic timing. Fat-soluble vitamins (A, D, E, and K) are best taken with meals containing fats for optimal absorption. Meanwhile, water-soluble vitamins (B vitamins and vitamin C) can be taken outside of meals, although taking them with food can help avoid stomach upset for some people.

Chapter 7: Nourishing Your Fasting Lifestyle

For electrolytes, timing can be more flexible; they can be consumed during fasting periods to maintain hydration and electrolyte balance, especially if you're active or live in a hot climate. Omega-3 supplements can be taken during eating windows to enhance absorption.

Consulting Healthcare Professionals

Before introducing any new supplement into your routine, a conversation with a healthcare provider is crucial. They can offer guidance tailored to your health history, dietary needs, and fasting practices, ensuring that any supplements you take support rather than detract from your health goals. This dialogue can also help prevent potential interactions between supplements and any medications you may be taking.

Bringing supplements into your intermittent fasting practice can enrich your nutritional landscape, ensuring your body receives a well-rounded array of nutrients necessary for optimal function. Through careful assessment of your needs, selecting the right supplements, mindful timing, and professional guidance, you can enhance your fasting experience, supporting your body's health and wellness goals.

As this chapter closes, we've navigated through the nuanced layers of integrating supplements into your fasting regimen, highlighting the importance of a holistic approach to nutrition. This exploration underscores the synergy between diet, supplementation, and fasting, each component playing a pivotal role in fostering a vibrant, healthy life. Moving forward, we'll continue to unravel the threads of a well-crafted fasting lifestyle, delving deeper into strategies and insights that empower you to live your healthiest life, one fasting window at a time.

Chapter 8: Smooth Sailing Through Fasting Challenges

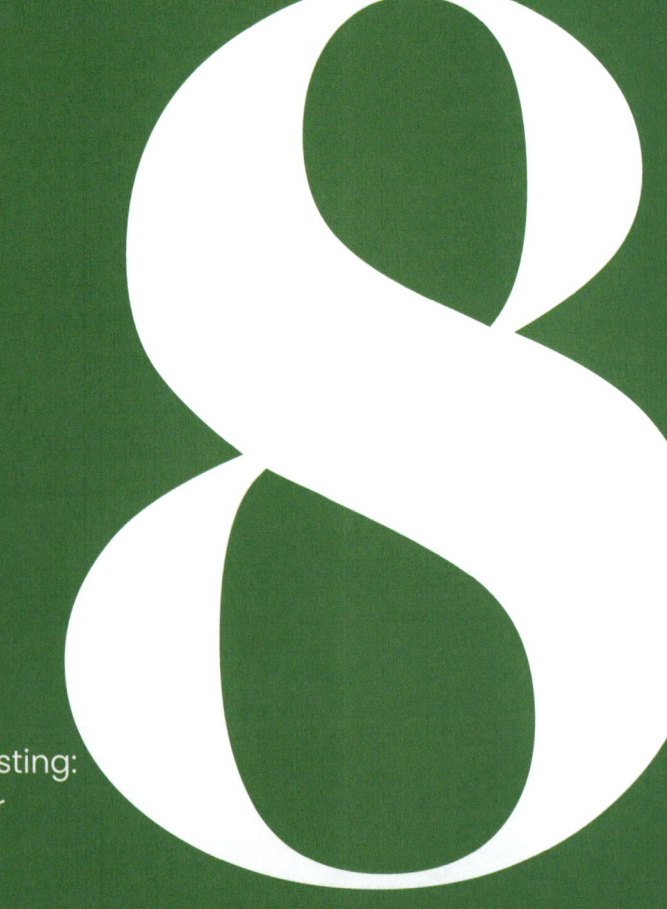

Intermittent Fasting: Transform Your Body and Mind

Chapter 8: Smooth Sailing Through Fasting Challenges

Imagine hitting a steep hill during a leisurely bike ride. You've been enjoying the breeze, the scenery, and the rhythm of pedalling on flat ground. Suddenly, this hill appears. It's unexpected, but not insurmountable. You adjust your gears, maybe slow down a bit, but you keep going. Before you know it, you're at the top, looking down at the path you conquered. That's a lot like intermittent fasting. You're cruising along when challenges like social pressures, scheduling conflicts, and initial hunger show up. They might slow you down, but they won't stop you. Here's how to adjust your gears and keep moving forward.

Identifying and Overcoming Common Fasting Challenges

- Social Pressures: Attending a family gathering or a dinner out with friends where food is a central feature can test your resolve. Prepare in advance by planning your fasting schedule around these events when possible. If you're in your fasting period, sipping on sparkling water and engaging in conversations can keep you integrated without needing to eat. Explaining your fasting regimen to close friends and family can also garner support, making social situations more manageable.

- Scheduling Conflicts: Life's unpredictability can throw your fasting schedule off balance. Maybe your work shifts change, or a last-minute appointment means you can't eat within your usual window. The key is flexibility. Adjusting your eating window by an hour or two to accommodate changes can maintain the rhythm of intermittent fasting without causing undue stress.

- Initial Hunger: The first few days or weeks of intermittent fasting might come with hunger pangs as your body adjusts. Drinking plenty of water, herbal teas, or even coffee can help manage these. Also, keeping busy with activities like walking, reading, or practising a hobby can distract you until your next eating window opens.

Staying Motivated During Tough Times

Motivation can wane, especially when results seem slow or challenges keep coming. Here are a few strategies to keep your spirits up:

- Set small, achievable goals. Instead of focusing solely on the end goal, celebrate smaller milestones like completing a week of consistent fasting.
- Document your progress. Keeping a journal or taking pictures can provide visual proof of your journey and motivate you to keep going.
- Remind yourself of your 'why'. Reflecting on the reasons you started intermittent fasting can reignite your motivation.

Seeking Support When Needed

- Fasting Communities: Online forums, social media groups, or local meetups can connect you with others on similar paths. Sharing experiences, tips, and encouragement can make your fasting journey feel less lonely.
- Friends and Family: Don't underestimate the power of support from loved ones. Even if they're not fasting with you, their understanding and encouragement can be a strong motivator.
- Healthcare Professionals: If you're facing medical or nutritional challenges related to fasting, consulting with a dietitian or doctor knowledgeable about intermittent fasting can provide personalised guidance.

Visual Element: The Fasting Challenge Compass

Imagine a compass, but instead of north, south, east, and west, the directions are labelled with common fasting challenges: Social Pressures, Scheduling Conflicts, Initial Hunger, and Waning Motivation. Each direction points towards a tip or strategy to navigate the challenge, serving as a quick reference or reminder that there's always a way to adjust and keep moving forward.

Chapter 8: Smooth Sailing Through Fasting Challenges

Intermittent fasting, like any lifestyle change, comes with its set of hills to climb. Recognizing these challenges as part of the process allows you to prepare and strategize effectively. With each challenge you overcome, you not only get closer to your goals but also build resilience and flexibility that benefit all areas of your life. Remember, it's not about never facing obstacles but about learning to navigate them with grace.

8.2 Breaking Through Weight Loss Plateaus

When the scale stops moving, it can feel like your hard work is no longer paying off. Hitting a weight loss plateau is a common part of the process, but it doesn't have to mean the end of your progress. Understanding why these plateaus happen, and how to push past them, can help you continue on your path to success.

Understanding Weight Loss Plateaus

A weight loss plateau occurs when your body adapts to your current diet and exercise routine, resulting in a halt in weight loss. Initially, your body responds to your new eating patterns and physical activities by shedding pounds. However, as you lose weight, your body requires fewer calories to function than it did at your heavier weight. This adjustment can lead to a balance between calorie intake and expenditure, causing your weight loss to stall. Recognizing a plateau as a sign that your body has adapted to your current regimen can be the first step in overcoming it.

Adjusting Your Fasting Regimen

One effective strategy to move past a plateau is to adjust your fasting regimen. If your body has grown accustomed to your current fasting schedule, changing it can jumpstart your metabolism. Consider these adjustments:

- Alter Fasting Durations: If you've been following a 16/8 method, try extending your fast to 18 hours or experimenting with 24-hour fasts once or twice a week.

- Vary Fasting Days: Instead of fasting every day, you might switch to alternate-day fasting or adopt a 5:2 schedule, fasting two days a week.
- Time Restructuring: Shift your eating window. If you usually break your fast in the morning, try waiting until noon or later, which can alter how your body utilises energy.

These changes can help your body out of its comfort zone, encouraging it to resume weight loss.

Reevaluating Caloric Intake and Expenditure

Another critical aspect of overcoming a weight loss plateau involves a careful look at both sides of the energy balance equation: calories in versus calories out. Here's how to tackle this:

- Track Your Intake: Use a food diary app to log everything you consume. You might find you're eating more calories than you realised, which can contribute to the plateau.
- Assess Your Nutrient Balance: Ensure your diet is rich in proteins, fibres, and healthy fats, which can influence satiety and metabolic rate. Sometimes, the quality of calories can be as important as the quantity.
- Increase Physical Activity: Boosting your exercise intensity or duration can help increase your calorie expenditure. Incorporate strength training to build muscle, which burns more calories at rest compared to fat.
- Mind Your NEAT: Non-exercise activity thermogenesis (NEAT), or the calories you burn through non-exercise movements like walking, gardening, or even fidgeting, can add up. Look for opportunities to move more throughout your day.

By carefully managing your calorie intake and increasing your calorie burn, you can tip the scales in favour of weight loss.

Chapter 8: Smooth Sailing Through Fasting Challenges

Patience and Persistence

Above all, patience and persistence are your best allies in overcoming a weight loss plateau. It's natural to feel frustrated when progress stalls, but remember, weight loss is not always linear. There will be ups and downs, and plateaus are just part of the journey. Keep focused on your long-term goals rather than getting too caught up in day-to-day fluctuations. Celebrate the changes in your body composition and health markers, such as improved blood sugar levels or lower blood pressure, even if the scale isn't moving. Sometimes, the most significant transformations are happening in places you can't measure with a scale.

Remember, overcoming a weight loss plateau is possible with strategic adjustments and a commitment to your goals. By understanding why plateaus happen, tweaking your fasting regimen, reassessing your caloric balance, and staying the course, you can continue making strides toward your weight loss objectives.

8.3 Dealing with Hunger Pangs and Cravings

Navigating the waters of intermittent fasting often means encountering the dual challenges of hunger pangs and cravings. Recognizing the nuances between these two experiences is the first step in managing them effectively. Hunger pangs signal the body's need for nourishment, while cravings are a complex mix of emotional and physiological cues driving us toward specific foods, often for reasons unrelated to actual hunger.

Differentiating Between Hunger and Cravings

Understanding the distinction between hunger and cravings lays the foundation for a successful fasting experience. Hunger is a physical sensation, a gentle reminder from our body that it's time to refuel. It builds gradually and can be satisfied with a variety of foods. Cravings, conversely, are acute desires for particular foods and are often tied to emotional states or external cues rather than genuine hunger.

Recognizing this difference empowers you to respond appropriately, feeding your body when it needs nourishment and addressing the root causes of cravings without derailing your fasting goals.

Natural Remedies for Managing Hunger

When hunger strikes, especially during your fasting window, there are several natural strategies you can employ to ease the sensation without breaking your fast:

- Stay Hydrated: Sometimes, our bodies confuse thirst with hunger. Drinking a glass of water or herbal tea can alleviate what feels like hunger pangs, keeping you on track until your next meal.
- Practice Mindfulness: Taking a moment to breathe deeply and focus on the present can help you ride out the wave of hunger. Mindfulness practices encourage a connection with your body, helping distinguish between true hunger and the desire to eat out of habit or boredom.
- Engage in Light Activity: A brief walk, some gentle stretching, or a low-intensity activity can shift your focus from hunger and help the feeling pass.

Healthy Ways to Satisfy Cravings

Cravings can be persistent, but with a few strategies, you can satisfy them in a manner that aligns with your fasting schedule and nutritional goals:

- Choose Healthier Alternatives: If you're craving something sweet, opt for fresh fruit like berries or an apple. Craving crunch? Try raw vegetables with a sprinkle of sea salt or a dash of vinegar for flavour.
- Portion Control: If you decide to indulge in what you're craving, do so in moderation. A small piece of dark chocolate or a single

Chapter 8: Smooth Sailing Through Fasting Challenges

serving of chips can satisfy your craving without leading to overindulgence.

- Timing Is Key: Incorporate a craved item into your meals, not as an extra snack. Adding a small portion of dark chocolate to your lunch, for example, lets you enjoy the treat without extra calories outside your eating window.

Preventing Cravings

The most effective way to handle cravings is to prevent them before they start. This proactive approach involves:

- Balanced Meals: Ensuring your meals are well-rounded with a good mix of proteins, fats, and carbohydrates helps keep blood sugar levels stable, reducing the likelihood of cravings.
- Regular Eating Schedule: Eating at consistent times during your eating window can help regulate your body's hunger signals, making unexpected cravings less likely.
- Mindful Eating: Paying attention to your meals, savouring each bite, and avoiding distractions while eating can increase meal satisfaction, making cravings for more, or different, food less compelling.
- Sufficient Sleep: Lack of sleep can disrupt hormonal balance, leading to increased hunger and cravings. Prioritising a full night's rest can help keep these urges in check.

By understanding and implementing these strategies, you equip yourself with the tools needed to distinguish between hunger and cravings, address them healthfully, and, when possible, avoid them altogether. This knowledge not only supports your fasting efforts but also enhances your overall relationship with food, leading to a more balanced and fulfilling approach to eating.

8.4 Adjusting Your Fasting Schedule for Maximum Benefit

In the dynamic dance of life, where routines ebb and flow like the tide, a rigid fasting schedule might not always harmonise with our changing rhythms. Recognizing when and how to modify your fasting plan can turn potential disruptions into opportunities for enhanced health and well-being. This segment guides you through refining your fasting practice, ensuring it remains a supportive and fluid part of your daily life.

Evaluating Your Current Fasting Schedule

Before you tweak your fasting schedule, taking a moment to assess its current impact on your lifestyle and health is crucial. Here are several indicators to consider:

- Energy Levels: Do you feel energised or lethargic during fasting and eating windows? An ideal schedule should boost your energy rather than deplete it.
- Sleep Quality: Has your sleep improved or worsened since starting your fasting regimen? Proper rest is vital for the body's recovery and overall health.
- Physical Performance: For those who exercise, does your fasting schedule support or hinder your workouts? The timing of your fasting should align with your physical activity for optimal performance and recovery.
- Hunger and Cravings: Are hunger and cravings manageable, or do they feel overwhelming? Your fasting schedule might need adjustments if you're constantly battling hunger.
- Mood and Focus: Consider whether your mood and focus have improved or if you're experiencing irritability and difficulty concentrating. Fasting should enhance mental clarity, not detract from it.

Chapter 8: Smooth Sailing Through Fasting Challenges

After this assessment, you'll have a clearer picture of how your current fasting schedule aligns with your health goals and lifestyle, providing a foundation for making informed adjustments.

Flexibility in Fasting

Adaptability is key in maintaining a fasting regimen that complements your life rather than complicates it. Life is replete with unexpected events, from last-minute work assignments to family gatherings, all of which can disrupt a rigid fasting schedule. Here's how to embrace flexibility:

- Adjust for Special Occasions: If a celebration falls during your fasting window, consider shifting your eating window to partake in the event. Resuming your regular schedule afterwards minimises disruption to your routine.
- Listen to Your Body: Some days, your body may need more nourishment due to increased physical activity or stress. Allowing yourself to eat earlier or extend your eating window on these days respects your body's needs.
- Plan for Busy Days: On particularly hectic days, a shorter fasting window might be more manageable and prevent you from feeling overwhelmed.

This adaptable approach ensures your fasting regimen supports your lifestyle, making it a sustainable practice rather than a source of stress.

Experimenting With New Fasting Windows

Exploring different fasting durations and times can uncover a schedule that resonates better with your body and routines. Here's a safe way to experiment:

- Start Small: If you're considering extending your fasting period, do so in small increments to allow your body to adjust gradually.

- Track Your Experience: Keep a journal of how you feel, changes in energy levels, and any other noteworthy effects as you try different fasting windows.
- Give It Time: Allow at least a few weeks to truly gauge how a new fasting schedule works for you. Immediate shifts in how you feel may not fully reflect long-term effects.

This methodical approach to experimentation respects your body's adaptation process and helps identify a fasting rhythm that enhances your health and fits your lifestyle.

Monitoring and Adjusting Based on Results

Continuous monitoring of your fasting regimen's effects on your health and well-being allows for ongoing optimization. Here are some strategies:

- Use Health Apps: Leveraging apps to track fasting hours, caloric intake, and even mood and sleep quality can provide valuable insights into how different schedules affect you.
- Regular Health Check-ups: Periodic check-ups and blood tests can reveal the physiological impacts of your fasting regimen, guiding further adjustments.
- Reflect Regularly: Set aside time each month to reflect on your fasting experience. Consider what's working and what might need changing based on your goals, health, and lifestyle.

This vigilant approach to monitoring ensures that your fasting schedule remains aligned with your evolving health needs and life circumstances, allowing for adjustments that keep your regimen effective and beneficial.

In weaving these strategies into the fabric of your fasting practice, you cultivate a responsive and dynamic approach that honours your body's needs, accommodates life's unpredictability, and supports your health goals. This fluidity in managing your fasting schedule not only enhances its benefits but also ensures it remains a positive and enriching part of your life, seamlessly integrated with the rhythms of your daily existence.

8.5 Emotional Eating and Fasting: Strategies for Success

Navigating the waters of intermittent fasting means not only managing physical hunger but also understanding the complex interplay between our emotions and eating habits. Emotional eating—the act of turning to food for comfort, stress relief, or as a reward—presents a unique set of challenges, especially when it disrupts fasting schedules or leads to overindulgence. Recognizing the triggers of emotional eating, developing healthier coping mechanisms, integrating mindfulness into your eating habits, and seeking professional support when necessary are pivotal steps in fostering a successful fasting experience.

Recognizing Emotional Eating Triggers

The first step toward addressing emotional eating is to pinpoint the emotions that prompt you to reach for food. These can range from stress and boredom to sadness and loneliness. It's crucial to observe patterns in your behaviour: Do you find yourself in the kitchen after a stressful day at work? Do you snack endlessly when you're bored, even if you're not truly hungry? Identifying these patterns allows you to anticipate and intercept emotional eating before it starts.

- Keep a food and mood diary: Jot down what you eat, when, and how you're feeling at the time. Over time, you'll start to see connections between your emotions and food intake.
- Reflect on your history with food: Sometimes, our relationship with food is deeply rooted in our past. Understanding this relationship can shed light on current emotional eating habits.

Developing Healthier Coping Mechanisms

Once you've identified the emotions driving you to eat, the next step is finding alternative ways to cope. Replacing emotional eating with healthier habits can help you maintain your fasting schedule and improve your overall well-being.

- Get moving: Physical activity is a powerful stress reliever. Whether it's a brisk walk, a yoga session, or a dance class, find an activity you enjoy that gets you moving.
- Explore hobbies: Engaging in hobbies or learning something new can distract from the urge to eat and fill your time with rewarding, fulfilling activities.
- Connect with others: Sometimes, all we need is a listening ear. Reach out to friends or family members when you're feeling down or stressed instead of turning to the pantry.
- Practice relaxation techniques: Deep breathing, meditation, and progressive muscle relaxation are effective tools for managing stress and emotional upheaval.

Integrating Mindfulness into Eating

Mindful eating encourages you to slow down and truly experience your food—its taste, texture, and how it makes you feel. This practice can help you recognize true hunger from emotional hunger, making it easier to stick to your fasting and eating windows.

- Eat without distractions: Turn off the TV, put down your phone, and focus solely on your meal. This helps you tune into your body's hunger and satiety signals.
- Savour each bite: Take the time to chew your food thoroughly and appreciate its flavours and textures. This can increase meal satisfaction and prevent overeating.
- Check-in with your hunger: Before eating, ask yourself if you're truly hungry or if you're reaching for food in response to an emotion. If it's the latter, refer to your list of alternative coping mechanisms.

Seeking Professional Support

For some, emotional eating is deeply ingrained and challenging to overcome alone. If you find that emotional eating persists despite your best efforts, it may be time to seek support from a mental health professional. Therapists or counsellors specialising in eating behaviours can provide the tools and strategies to address the root causes of emotional eating.

- Look for a therapist with experience in eating disorders or emotional eating. They can offer tailored strategies that address your specific challenges.
- Consider group therapy or support groups. Sharing your experiences with others facing similar struggles can provide comfort, insights, and additional strategies for managing emotional eating.
- Explore cognitive-behavioural therapy (CBT). CBT is particularly effective for changing negative thought patterns and behaviours related to emotional eating.

Successfully managing emotional eating requires a multifaceted approach: recognizing triggers, replacing the habit with healthier coping mechanisms, practising mindful eating, and seeking support when needed. By addressing the emotional aspect of eating, you can better navigate the challenges of intermittent fasting, ensuring that your relationship with food supports not just your physical health, but your emotional well-being too.

8.6 Reevaluating Goals and Making Sustainable Changes

In the flow of life, where intermittent fasting becomes part of the daily rhythm, setting and revisiting goals ensures that your commitment remains aligned with your evolving aspirations and realities. Like a tree that adjusts its growth towards the light, so too must your fasting practice flex and grow towards your personal light—your well-being and satisfaction.

The Importance of Realistic Goal-Setting

At the heart of a fulfilling fasting experience lies the art of crafting goals that are as realistic as they are inspiring. Goals that stretch too far may lead to disappointment, while those set too low might not offer enough challenge to motivate. Finding that sweet spot involves understanding your current lifestyle, acknowledging your strengths and challenges, and setting aims that encourage but don't overwhelm you. For instance, if you're new to fasting, aiming to fast every day might set you up for stress; starting with a few days a week can offer a gentle introduction, allowing for adjustment and growth.

Adjusting Goals as You Progress

Life is not static, and neither are you. As you move through your fasting journey, it's vital to pause and reflect on your progress. Have you achieved the goals you set? Have circumstances in your life changed, altering your ability to meet those targets? Adjusting your goals doesn't signify failure; it's a recognition of your dynamic nature and life's unpredictability. Perhaps you started fasting with weight loss in mind but discovered a passion for improved energy and mental clarity along the way. Shifting your focus to these new-found benefits keeps your practice relevant and rewarding.

Making Intermittent Fasting a Lifestyle

For intermittent fasting to weave seamlessly into the fabric of your life, viewing it through the lens of lifestyle rather than a temporary diet is key. This perspective shift encourages you to find joy and fulfilment in the process, integrating fasting into your life in ways that feel natural and sustainable. This might mean aligning your fasting schedule with your work life, social commitments, and exercise routine, making adjustments as these elements of your life ebb and flow. The aim is to blend fasting into your daily existence so that it enhances rather than complicates your life.

Chapter 8: Smooth Sailing Through Fasting Challenges

Celebrating Non-Scale Victories

While the scale might be the most obvious measure of progress, the true richness of intermittent fasting is found in the tapestry of non-scale victories. These might be the subtle but profound changes you experience, such as waking up feeling rested, finding joy in healthier food choices, or noticing a new-found steadiness in your mood and energy levels throughout the day. Celebrating these milestones reminds you that intermittent fasting's value lies not just in pounds lost but in the enhanced quality of life gained. Recognizing and valuing these victories fuels your motivation and commitment, highlighting the holistic benefits of your fasting journey.

As this chapter draws to a close, remember that the path of intermittent fasting is one of exploration and growth. Setting realistic goals, adjusting them as you evolve, integrating fasting into your life in a way that brings joy, and celebrating all forms of progress ensures that your fasting practice is a rewarding and enriching part of your journey towards health and well-being. These principles not only guide your fasting journey but also offer a blueprint for approaching life's other aspirations with flexibility, resilience, and a focus on holistic success.

In the next chapter, we'll continue to build on these foundations, exploring strategies to deepen your fasting practice and enhance your overall quality of life.

Chapter 9: Mind Over Meal: Fostering a Positive Fasting Mindset

Chapter 9: Mind Over Meal: Fostering a Positive Fasting Mindset

Picture this: You're at a buffet, your plate in hand, surrounded by an array of foods from every corner of the globe. The choices seem endless, but instead of diving right in, you pause. You're not just thinking about what appeals to your taste buds but also how it fits into your fasting schedule. This moment of pause, this decision to choose mindfully over mindlessly, encapsulates the essence of fostering a positive mindset around fasting. It's not just about what you eat or when you eat—it's about changing your relationship with food, one thoughtful choice at a time.

Embracing Change and Challenge

Change isn't easy, especially when it involves rethinking a fundamental part of our lives like eating. Yet, embracing change is crucial for growth. When you start fasting, view it not as giving something up but as gaining a new perspective on your health and habits. Here's a real-life scenario many can relate to: Sunday family dinners, a tradition where food is abundant and the atmosphere is jovial. In the past, you might have indulged without a second thought. Now, with fasting, you approach these gatherings differently, choosing your dishes more thoughtfully, savouring each bite, and finding that your enjoyment of the meal deepens. This shift in perspective is a powerful testament to the growth that comes from embracing change.

Mindfulness and Fasting

Mindfulness, the practice of being present and fully engaged with whatever we're doing at the moment, can transform your fasting experience. Imagine you're starting your fasting window, and suddenly, you're hit with a craving for something sweet. Instead of reacting impulsively, you pause. You take a deep breath, acknowledge the craving without judgement, and remind yourself why you chose to fast. This moment of mindfulness allows the craving to pass without breaking your fast. It's a small victory, but over time, these moments add up, strengthening your fasting practice.

- Exercise: Next time you eat, try this mindfulness exercise: Turn off all distractions. Before you take your first bite, take a moment to appreciate the colours and smells of your food. Chew slowly, noticing the textures and flavours. Reflect on how the food makes you feel, both physically and emotionally. This simple practice can deepen your appreciation for food and enhance your fasting mindset.

Overcoming Mental Barriers

Resistance is part of the human experience, especially when trying something new like fasting. Common hurdles include the fear of feeling hungry, concerns about not having enough energy, and the worry of missing out on social eating occasions. Overcoming these barriers starts with education—understanding that hunger comes in waves and that our bodies are well-equipped to handle short periods without food. Energy levels can increase due to the body tapping into fat stores for fuel. As for social occasions, they become opportunities to practise flexibility within your fasting regimen, finding a balance between social enjoyment and your fasting goals.

- Checklist:
    - ☐ Research the benefits and mechanics of intermittent fasting.
    - ☐ Remind yourself of your reasons for fasting whenever you encounter resistance.
    - ☐ Plan for flexibility in your fasting schedule to accommodate special occasions.

Affirmations and Positive Self-talk

The words we say to ourselves have immense power. Positive affirmations and self-talk can be instrumental in reinforcing your commitment to fasting. Instead of thinking, "I can't eat until noon," reframe it as, "I'm choosing to nourish my body at noon." This subtle shift in language can make a significant difference in how you perceive fasting.

Chapter 9: Mind Over Meal: Fostering a Positive Fasting Mindset

- Affirmations to Try:
  - ☐ "I nourish my body with intention and mindfulness."
  - ☐ "Each fasting hour is a step towards my health goals."
  - ☐ "I embrace the strength and discipline fasting brings into my life."

Embedding these affirmations in your daily routine, perhaps by saying them out loud each morning or writing them in a journal, can bolster your resolve and keep you focused on the positive aspects of your fasting journey.

In weaving these threads of change, acceptance, mindfulness, mental resilience, and positive self-talk into the fabric of your fasting practice, you create a tapestry rich with personal growth, health, and fulfilment. This chapter isn't just about fasting; it's about transforming your relationship with food and yourself, one mindful choice at a time.

9.2 Visualisation and Goal Setting for Long-Term Success

Visualising your success with intermittent fasting is like picturing the top of a mountain before you begin your climb. It's about seeing the peak, feeling the triumph of reaching it, and understanding the path you'll take to get there. This mental image serves not just as motivation but as a map, guiding your actions and decisions along the way. When you close your eyes and envision how you'll feel, look, and live once you've integrated fasting into your life successfully, you solidify your commitment and enhance your clarity on why you're taking this path.

The Power of Visualization

Imagine the version of yourself that you want to become through intermittent fasting. Maybe you see yourself with more energy, participating in activities you love, or simply enjoying a sense of health you haven't felt in years. Holding this image in your mind strengthens your resolve on challenging days and reminds you why you started fasting in the first place. Here's how to harness visualisation effectively:

- Daily Visualization Practice: Spend a few minutes each morning or evening in quiet contemplation, picturing your fasting goals as already achieved. Focus on the feelings, the senses, and the experiences of this future you.
- Use Visual Cues: Surround yourself with images or objects that represent your goals. It could be pictures of healthy meals, workout plans, or even a piece of clothing you look forward to wearing comfortably.

Setting SMART Goals

To turn your visualisations into reality, your aspirations need structure. SMART goals break down your fasting ambitions into actionable steps. Here's what each letter stands for and how it applies to fasting:

- Specific: Define what you want to achieve with fasting. Is it weight loss, improved health markers, or enhanced mental clarity? Be as detailed as possible.
- Measurable: Attach numbers to your goals. How many pounds do you want to lose? What blood sugar level are you aiming for? This makes it easier to track progress.
- Achievable: Ensure your goals are realistic given your current lifestyle, health status, and commitments. Setting the bar at a sensible height keeps motivation high.
- Relevant: Your fasting goals should align with your broader life ambitions. If you're aiming for a more active lifestyle, consider how fasting will fuel your energy levels and physical recovery.
- Time-bound: Give yourself a deadline. Having a target date adds urgency and helps prioritise actions and decisions related to your fasting practice.

Chapter 9: Mind Over Meal: Fostering a Positive Fasting Mindset

Creating a Vision Board

A vision board serves as a daily visual reminder of your fasting goals and the life you're working towards. Here's how to create one that inspires you:

- Collect Images and Quotes: Look for pictures that represent your fasting goals, such as healthy foods, exercise routines, or serene spaces for meditation. Add motivational quotes that resonate with you.
- Choose a Format: Decide whether you prefer a digital vision board that you can keep on your phone or computer, or a physical one that you can place in a visible spot in your home.
- Arrange and Display: Organise your collected items in a way that appeals to you and place your vision board somewhere you'll see it daily. Let it be a constant source of inspiration and encouragement.

Adjusting Goals Over Time

As you progress with intermittent fasting, your initial goals might need some tweaking. Maybe you've surpassed your weight loss target ahead of schedule, or you've discovered new health benefits that shift your focus. It's important to periodically reassess and adjust your goals to reflect where you are now and where you want to go next. Consider this a sign of growth rather than a setback. Flexibility ensures your fasting practice evolves with you, remaining both challenging and rewarding. To do this:

- Regular Check-ins: Set aside time every month to review your goals. What's working? What's not? Are there new objectives you want to pursue?
- Seek Feedback: Sometimes, an outside perspective can offer valuable insights. Talk to friends, family, or a health professional about your progress and potential areas for adjustment.

- Celebrate Progress: Recognize and reward yourself for the milestones you've achieved. This reinforces positive behaviour and sets the stage for further success.

Through visualisation, SMART goals, a personalised vision board, and the flexibility to adjust your aims, you lay down a solid foundation for long-term success in your fasting practice. Each element of this process not only keeps you aligned with your objectives but also deepens your connection to the journey, making every step forward meaningful and every achievement a cause for celebration.

9.3 The Role of Community and Support in Fasting

In the world of intermittent fasting, the path you walk can sometimes feel solitary. However, the strength found in unity and shared experiences can illuminate this path, making the journey not only more bearable but also more enriching. This section explores the invaluable role that community and support play in enhancing your fasting experience, offering practical advice on how to connect with like-minded individuals, and highlighting the profound impact of nurturing supportive relationships.

Finding Your Fasting Tribe

Locating a community of fellow fasters offers a treasure trove of resources, empathy, and encouragement. Here's how you might go about discovering your fasting tribe:

- Online Platforms: Digital forums and social media groups dedicated to intermittent fasting are plentiful. Platforms such as Reddit, Facebook, and dedicated fasting apps host vibrant communities where members share advice, success stories, and challenges. When joining these spaces, look for groups that match your specific interests within the fasting spectrum, whether it's the 16/8 method, OMAD (One Meal A Day), or extended fasting.

Chapter 9: Mind Over Meal: Fostering a Positive Fasting Mindset

- Local Meetups: While digital connections are invaluable, face-to-face interactions can deepen your sense of belonging. Websites like Meetup.com often list local groups dedicated to fasting and health. Attending these gatherings can provide a sense of camaraderie and accountability that's hard to replicate online.
- Fasting Events: Keep an eye out for workshops, talks, or conferences on fasting and nutrition. These events not only expand your knowledge but also provide networking opportunities with fellow fasting enthusiasts and experts.

The Importance of Supportive Relationships

The people closest to us—our friends and family—hold significant sway over our fasting experience. Their support can be a cornerstone of our success. Here's how to cultivate understanding and encouragement from them:

- Open Communication: Share your reasons for choosing to fast, focusing on the health benefits and personal growth you hope to achieve. Being open about your goals helps others understand your commitment and reduces the likelihood of unsupportive behaviour.
- Setting Boundaries: Politely set clear boundaries around food-related socialising. Suggest alternative activities that don't centre around meals, or propose gatherings during your eating window.
- Seek a Fasting Buddy: Encourage friends or family members to try fasting with you. Having a fasting buddy can significantly boost your motivation and provide a shared experience to bond over.

Learning from Others

The collective wisdom of a community can be a powerful tool in refining your fasting practice. Here's how to maximise learning from your fasting tribe:

- Share Stories: Engage actively in community discussions. Share your own experiences and listen to others. You might find someone who's navigated a challenge you're facing or discover a new strategy that enhances your fasting regimen.

- Ask for Advice: Don't hesitate to seek guidance from more experienced fasters. Most communities are eager to help newcomers. Whether you're struggling with hunger pangs or seeking recipe ideas for your eating window, there's likely someone who can offer insight.

- Stay Open-Minded: Every faster's experience is unique. Stay open to different perspectives and approaches. What works for one person may not for another, but understanding the breadth of fasting experiences can inspire you to experiment and find what works best for you.

Giving Back

As you gain experience and confidence in your fasting journey, consider giving back to the community that has supported you. Here's why sharing your journey can be rewarding:

- Inspiring Others: Your success stories can be a beacon of hope for those just starting or struggling. Sharing the highs and lows of your journey provides a realistic picture of what fasting entails, encouraging others to persevere.

- Offering Support: Remember the support you sought in your early days? Now's your chance to be that supportive voice for someone else. Providing encouragement, answering questions, and simply being there for others enriches the community and deepens your understanding and commitment to fasting.

- Creating Resources: If you've found particular strategies or tools beneficial, consider creating resources to share with the community. Whether it's a meal planning guide, a motivational podcast, or a blog documenting your journey, these contributions can become valuable assets for fellow fasters.

In the tapestry of intermittent fasting, the threads of community and support weave through, strengthening and embellishing the fabric of our experience. Through finding your tribe, fostering supportive relationships, learning from shared wisdom, and giving back, you not only enhance your fasting journey but also contribute to a collective journey, rich with growth, discovery, and mutual upliftment.

9.4 Celebrating Milestones and Navigating Setbacks

In the world of intermittent fasting, the road is marked with signs of both triumph and challenge. Recognizing and celebrating each win, no matter its size, is akin to watering the garden of your determination, allowing it to flourish. Conversely, encountering setbacks is not the end of the path but rather a twist in the journey, offering lessons and insights that can fuel your growth and resilience.

Recognizing and Celebrating Progress

The act of acknowledging your achievements serves as a powerful motivator, reinforcing your commitment to fasting and your broader health aspirations. Each milestone, from sticking to your fasting schedule for a full week to noticing increased energy levels, deserves recognition. Here are some strategies to celebrate your progress effectively:

- Create a Reward System: Tie specific milestones to rewards that complement your fasting goals. For instance, after a month of consistent fasting, treat yourself to a new workout outfit or a cooking class to explore healthier recipes.
- Share Your Achievements: Sometimes, the joy of reaching a milestone is amplified by sharing it with others. Whether it's with your fasting community, friends, or family, talking about your achievements can boost your confidence and inspire others.

- Reflect on Your Growth: Set aside time regularly to look back on how far you've come since you started fasting. Writing down your reflections can provide a tangible record of your progress, highlighting not just the changes in your body, but in your mindset and approach to health and wellness.

Constructive Handling of Setbacks

Setbacks are an inevitable part of any endeavour that requires change and discipline. Instead of viewing them as failures, interpret them as opportunities to learn and recalibrate. Here's how to navigate setbacks constructively:

- Identify the Cause: Take a step back and assess what led to the setback. Was it a change in routine, a particularly stressful week, or perhaps a lack of planning? Understanding the root cause can help you address it directly.
- Adjust Your Approach: Based on your assessment, you might need to tweak your fasting schedule, find new strategies to manage stress, or refine your meal planning process. Flexibility is key in finding what works best for you.
- Seek Support: Don't hesitate to reach out to your support network for advice, encouragement, or simply a listening ear. Sometimes, just talking about a setback can lessen its impact and help you find a way forward.

Maintaining Motivation Through Challenges

When faced with slow progress or unexpected obstacles, keeping your motivation intact is crucial. Here are some strategies to maintain your drive:

- Set Short-Term Goals: While having a long-term vision is important, short-term goals can provide immediate focus and a sense of achievement. These could be as simple as completing a 24-hour fast or trying a new healthy recipe.

Chapter 9: Mind Over Meal: Fostering a Positive Fasting Mindset

- Visual Reminders: Keep visual cues of your goals and progress in places you see daily. This could be a photo of yourself at a healthier time, a motivational quote, or a chart tracking your fasting days.
- Celebrate the Small Wins: Every step forward is a win, no matter how small. Did you resist a craving, or did you complete your fasting window despite a hectic day? Acknowledge and celebrate these moments.

The Role of Gratitude

Cultivating a sense of gratitude can transform your fasting experience from one of deprivation to one of abundance. Here's why gratitude matters and how to practise it:

- Focus on What You Have: Instead of dwelling on the foods or habits you might be missing, shift your focus to what you're gaining through fasting—whether it's better health, more energy, or a deeper connection with your body.
- Gratitude Journal: Keeping a gratitude journal specifically related to your fasting experience can help shift your perspective. Each day, write down three things related to fasting that you're grateful for, such as the ability to fast, the availability of healthy foods, or even the challenge itself, as it offers a chance to grow.
- Acknowledge Your Body's Efforts: Your body is your partner in this fasting journey. Take time to appreciate its resilience and the work it does to adapt and thrive under changing conditions.

In threading through the ups and downs of intermittent fasting, celebrating each milestone and navigating setbacks with a constructive mindset not only propels you forward but enriches your journey with growth and self-discovery. By maintaining motivation, even in the face of challenges, and cultivating gratitude for the journey and your body's capabilities, you lay the foundation for lasting change and a deeper appreciation for the process and its rewards.

9.5 Intermittent Fasting as a Path to Self-Discovery

The act of fasting goes beyond the mere abstention from food; it invites us into a deeper conversation with ourselves. This dialogue unveils the nuanced language of our body and mind, revealing insights that often go unnoticed amidst the clamour of daily routines. Through fasting, we not only learn to interpret these messages but also to respond in ways that nurture our growth and well-being.

Learning about Your Body and Mind

Fasting serves as a mirror, reflecting the intricacies of our physiological and psychological landscapes. It teaches us to discern the whisper of true hunger from the noise of cravings fueled by habit or emotion. This understanding encourages a more harmonious relationship with food, where choices are guided by nourishment rather than compulsion. Furthermore, fasting can illuminate our emotional relationship with eating, helping us to untangle the threads of comfort and sustenance. In this light, we learn that hunger is not an enemy but a natural rhythm of the body, a rhythm that, when listened to, can lead to optimal health and vitality.

- Observation Exercise: For one week, keep a log of your physical sensations and emotional states during fasting periods. Note any patterns or discoveries, such as specific times when hunger strikes or emotions that trigger the desire to eat. This exercise is not about judgement but about fostering awareness and understanding.

Fasting and Personal Growth

The discipline required for fasting often translates into other areas of life, instilling habits of perseverance and resilience. Each fasting window is a commitment to self-care, a testament to our ability to set

Chapter 9: Mind Over Meal: Fostering a Positive Fasting Mindset

boundaries and prioritise our well-being. This practice of self-discipline can spill over into career goals, personal projects, and relationships, empowering us to make conscious choices that align with our deepest values and aspirations. Moreover, fasting can be a catalyst for emotional resilience, teaching us to sit with discomfort, whether it be hunger or emotional upheaval, and to move through it with grace and awareness.

- Reflection Exercise: After a challenging fasting day, write down what made it difficult and how you coped. Reflect on how these coping strategies could be applied to other challenges in your life.

Embracing New Habits and Hobbies

The time and energy saved from meal planning, shopping, and eating can open doors to new pursuits. Fasting can give us moments to explore passions that have lain dormant, be they creative endeavours, physical activities, or intellectual pursuits. This exploration not only enriches our lives but also reinforces the benefits of fasting by filling the spaces left by old habits with fulfilling and life-affirming experiences.

- Try Something New: Use the time you would have spent on a meal to engage in an activity you've been curious about. It could be as simple as reading a book, taking a walk in nature, or starting a creative project. Notice how these activities impact your fasting experience.

The Transformative Power of Fasting

The journey of fasting is replete with moments of revelation and transformation. It invites a shift not just in how we eat but in how we live and relate to the world around us. As we align more closely with our body's natural rhythms and needs, we find ourselves moving through the world with greater intention and presence. This alignment fosters a sense of peace and contentment, illuminating the interconnectedness of our physical, mental, and emotional health. Furthermore, fasting can be a spiritual experience for some, offering a time of reflection, gratitude, and connection to something greater than ourselves. In these moments of quietude, we often find clarity and purpose, guiding lights on our path to self-discovery.

- Meditative Practice: During your next fast, dedicate a few moments to sit quietly, focusing on your breath. Allow thoughts and sensations to arise and pass without attachment. Use this time to reflect on your intentions for fasting and the values that guide your life. This practice can deepen the sense of connection to your inner self and the world around you.

The path of intermittent fasting, then, is much more than a dietary choice; it is a voyage into the depths of self-awareness and transformation. It challenges us to confront our habits, fears, and desires, offering a bridge to a more intentional and fulfilling way of being. Through this practice, we not only learn about the intricacies of our physical hunger but also about the hunger of our soul— for connection, growth, and a life lived in harmony with our deepest truths.

9.6 Looking Ahead: The Future of Your Fasting Journey

In the tapestry of life, where intermittent fasting weaves its intricate patterns, a mindset geared towards evolution and adaptability ensures that your practice grows alongside you. As each day unfurls, it brings with it a wealth of experiences and insights, shaping your approach to fasting and moulding it into a practice that resonates deeply with your evolving lifestyle and aspirations.

Evolving Your Fasting Practice

Imagine standing at the edge of a serene lake, your reflection clear against the calm waters. Just as the slightest breeze can alter this reflection, so too can life's changes ripple through your fasting practice. With each wave, you have the opportunity to adjust and refine your approach, ensuring it remains aligned with your current state of being and future goals.

Chapter 9: Mind Over Meal: Fostering a Positive Fasting Mindset

- Stay curious about new fasting research and methodologies, incorporating findings that resonate with you.
- Reflect on your routines and schedules, adjusting your fasting windows as your life shifts—be it a new job, a change in family dynamics, or simply a new season.
- Remember, your body's needs will change as you age, necessitating adjustments to your fasting regimen to maintain optimal health and vitality.

Lifelong Learning and Adaptation

Life is an unending journey of learning, and so too is the path of intermittent fasting. Keeping abreast of the latest in nutritional science and wellness not only enriches your understanding but also empowers you to make informed decisions about your fasting practice.

- Dedicate time each month to reading articles, listening to podcasts, or attending webinars focused on fasting, nutrition, and health.
- Experiment with integrating new foods, supplements, or eating patterns into your eating windows, noting how these changes impact your energy, mood, and overall well-being.
- View each adjustment not as a deviation from your path but as a step towards a more attuned and personalised fasting practice.

Anticipating Future Challenges

As with any endeavour worth pursuing, intermittent fasting comes with its set of challenges. Foreseeing these obstacles allows you to arm yourself with strategies to navigate them, ensuring they become stepping stones rather than stumbling blocks.

- Life events such as holidays, travel, or periods of stress can disrupt your fasting schedule. Planning ahead and allowing yourself flexibility during these times can help maintain your commitment without adding undue stress.

- Changes in health status may require modifications to your fasting practice. Regular check-ins with healthcare professionals ensure your fasting regimen supports your health at all stages.
- Social settings will continue to test your resolve. Cultivating a strong sense of self-assurance in your fasting choices empowers you to navigate social pressures with confidence.

Envisioning Your Future Self

Close your eyes for a moment and picture yourself in the future, thriving with the benefits that your dedicated fasting practice has cultivated. This vision of your future self is not just a dream but a potential reality that you are actively working towards.

- Take time regularly to visualise your goals as already achieved, feeling the emotions and physical sensations associated with this future state of health and fulfilment.
- Use this vision as a compass, guiding your choices and actions in the present to align with the future you aspire to.
- Let this picture of your future self be a beacon during times of doubt or difficulty, reminding you of the rewards that await your persistent efforts.

In the dance of life, where rhythms change and melodies shift, your fasting practice is both a partner and a guide. It evolves with you, adapting to the music of your life, ensuring that with each step, you move closer to a state of health, vitality, and fulfilment. The journey ahead is rich with potential, paved with lessons to learn, challenges to overcome, and triumphs to celebrate.

As we wrap up this exploration into the future of your fasting journey, remember that the essence of this practice lies in its fluidity and capacity for adaptation. It's a reflection of life itself—ever-changing, endlessly fascinating, and profoundly rewarding. The insights you've gained, the strategies you've armed yourself with, and the vision you

Chapter 9: Mind Over Meal: Fostering a Positive Fasting Mindset

carry for your future self set the stage for a journey that transcends the mere act of fasting to touch on the very art of living well.

In the chapters that follow, we'll continue to build on this foundation, exploring new dimensions of wellness and self-discovery, each step guided by the principles of mindfulness, adaptability, and a deep-rooted commitment to nurturing your best self.

CONCLUSION

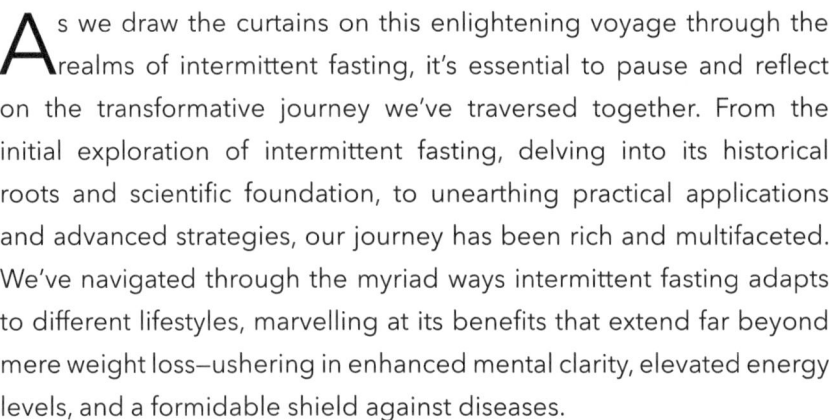

As we draw the curtains on this enlightening voyage through the realms of intermittent fasting, it's essential to pause and reflect on the transformative journey we've traversed together. From the initial exploration of intermittent fasting, delving into its historical roots and scientific foundation, to unearthing practical applications and advanced strategies, our journey has been rich and multifaceted. We've navigated through the myriad ways intermittent fasting adapts to different lifestyles, marvelling at its benefits that extend far beyond mere weight loss—ushering in enhanced mental clarity, elevated energy levels, and a formidable shield against diseases.

The key takeaways from our shared expedition cannot be overstated. Understanding the signals your body dispatches, the indispensability of a supportive community, the invigorating power of a positive mindset, and the criticality of setting realistic goals have emerged as pillars of a successful intermittent fasting practice. Our holistic approach—marrying intermittent fasting with adequate sleep, regular exercise, and effective stress management—promises a balanced and enriching lifestyle.

For middle-aged men and women, intermittent fasting unfurls as a beacon of hope, adeptly addressing age-related metabolic shifts and hormonal changes. It stands as a stalwart ally in managing weight, maintaining hormonal equilibrium, and bolstering overall well-being through the midlife transitions of menopause and andropause.

Conclusion

I implore you, dear readers, to embrace intermittent fasting not merely as a fleeting diet but as a lifelong journey of discovery and adaptation. I encourage you to embark on this path with a spirit of experimentation and flexibility, tuning into your body's unique rhythms and needs. Remember, patience and persistence are your companions as you navigate the myriad fasting methods to uncover what resonates with you.

The realm of intermittent fasting and nutrition is ever-evolving, brimming with new research and insights. Stay voracious for knowledge, keeping your mind open to refining your fasting practice as new information comes to light. Your journey doesn't end here; let curiosity be your guide as you continue to explore the vast landscapes of health and well-being.

I urge you to not walk this path in solitude but to share your journey—your triumphs, your setbacks, and everything in between. Whether through social media, support groups, or online communities, your story can be a source of inspiration and motivation, not just for you but for countless others embarking on their fasting journeys.

In closing, I extend my heartfelt gratitude to you for allowing me to be a part of your journey into the transformative world of intermittent fasting. It is my sincere hope that the insights shared within these pages serve as a beacon, guiding you towards a healthier, more vibrant existence. Approach your fasting journey with optimism, resilience, and an open heart, for the path ahead is replete with promise and potential.

Together, let's continue to explore, adapt, and thrive.

Yours in health and discovery,

Ry Shimanski

REFERENCES

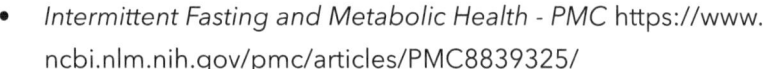

- *Intermittent Fasting and Metabolic Health - PMC* https://www.ncbi.nlm.nih.gov/pmc/articles/PMC8839325/
- *Effect of Intermittent Fasting on Reproductive Hormone ...* https://www.ncbi.nlm.nih.gov/pmc/articles/PMC9182756/
- *Fasting Through the Ages: Benefits of Ancient Practice* https://www.miragenews.com/fasting-through-the-ages-benefits-of-ancient-987227/
- *The Beneficial and Adverse Effects of Autophagic ...* https://www.ncbi.nlm.nih.gov/pmc/articles/PMC10509423/
- *Research on intermittent fasting shows health benefits* https://www.nia.nih.gov/news/research-intermittent-fasting-shows-health-benefits
- *16/8 Intermittent Fasting: Meal Plan, Benefits, and More* https://www.healthline.com/nutrition/16-8-intermittent-fasting
- *Eat Stop Eat Review: Does It Work for Weight Loss?* https://www.healthline.com/nutrition/eat-stop-eat-review
- *A randomised controlled trial of the 5:2 diet - PMC* https://www.ncbi.nlm.nih.gov/pmc/articles/PMC8598045/
- *Intermittent Fasting: What is it, and how does it work?* https://www.hopkinsmedicine.org/health/wellness-and-prevention/intermittent-fasting-what-is-it-and-how-does-it-work

References

- *SMART goals for fasting | Diet Doctor* https://www.dietdoctor.com/wp-content/uploads/2020/11/IF-SMART-goals-for-fasting-.pdf
- *Intermittent Fasting Supplements - Fullscript* https://fullscript.com/blog/taking-supplements-while-fasting#:~:text=Taking%20certain%20dietary%20supplements%20may,fatty%20acids%2C%20and%20soluble%20fiber.
- *The Fasting Method ~ Intermittent Fasting for Weight Loss* https://www.thefastingmethod.com/
- *Intermittent Fasting: What is it, and how does it work?* https://www.hopkinsmedicine.org/health/wellness-and-prevention/intermittent-fasting-what-is-it-and-how-does-it-work
- *The Benefits of Intermittent Fasting for Sleep* https://www.sleepfoundation.org/physical-health/intermittent-fasting-sleep
- *Intermittent fasting and exercise: How to do it safely* https://www.medicalnewstoday.com/articles/intermittent-fasting-and-working-out
- *Mindful Eating | The Nutrition Source | Harvard T.H. Chan ...* https://www.hsph.harvard.edu/nutritionsource/mindful-eating/
- *Effects of intermittent fasting on cognitive health and ...* https://academic.oup.com/nutritionreviews/article/81/9/1225/7116310
- *Autophagy in healthy ageing and disease* https://www.nature.com/articles/s43587-021-00098-4
- *How fasting can reduce disease risk by lowering inflammation* https://www.medicalnewstoday.com/articles/how-fasting-can-reduce-disease-risk-by-lowering-inflammation

- *Eat less, live longer? The science of fasting and longevity* https://gero.usc.edu/2019/04/18/eat-less-live-longer-the-science-of-fasting-and-longevity/
- *Is Intermittent Fasting Healthy for Women?* https://health.clevelandclinic.org/intermittent-fasting-for-women
- *Is Intermittent Fasting Healthy for Women?* https://health.clevelandclinic.org/intermittent-fasting-for-women
- *What Midlife Women Should Know About Intermittent Fasting* https://www.everydayhealth.com/womens-health/what-midlife-women-should-know-about-intermittent-fasting/
- *Intermittent fasting can help manage metabolic disease* https://www.endocrine.org/news-and-advocacy/news-room/2021/intermittent-fasting-can-help-manage-metabolic-disease
- *16/8 Intermittent Fasting: Meal Plan, Benefits, and ...* https://www.healthline.com/nutrition/16-8-intermittent-fasting
- *16/8 Intermittent Fasting: Meal Plan, Benefits, and More* https://www.healthline.com/nutrition/16-8-intermittent-fasting
- *Your Intermittent Fasting Meal Prep Guide* https://www.womansworld.com/posts/diet/intermittent-fasting-meal-prep-guide
- *What Fasting Supplements Should You Take and Why?* https://healthnews.com/nutrition/vitamins-and-supplements/what-fasting-supplements-should-you-take-and-why/
- *Intermittent Fasting: What is it, and how does it work?* https://www.hopkinsmedicine.org/health/wellness-and-prevention/intermittent-fasting-what-is-it-and-how-does-it-work
- *Challenges and solutions in intermittent fasting* https://thefast800.com/challenges-and-solutions-in-intermittent-fasting/
- *How Intermittent Fasting Affects Your Brain Health - ZOE* https://zoe.com/learn/intermittent-fasting-and-brain-health

References

- *Traditional and Medical Applications of Fasting - PMC* https://www.ncbi.nlm.nih.gov/pmc/articles/PMC8838777/
- *Intermittent Fasting: What is it, and how does it work?* https://www.hopkinsmedicine.org/health/wellness-and-prevention/intermittent-fasting-what-is-it-and-how-does-it-w ork
- *Mindfulness training can boost heart-healthy eating* https://www.nih.gov/news-events/nih-research-matters/mindfulness-training-can-boost-heart-healthy-eating
- *Fasting: The History, Pathophysiology and Complications* https://www.ncbi.nlm.nih.gov/pmc/articles/PMC1274154/
- *LCHF Living & Intermittent Fasting Support Group* https://connect.mayoclinic.org/group/lchf-living-intermittent-fasting/

Made in the USA
Columbia, SC
20 June 2024